The Ultimate Guide to Anal Sex for Women

SECOND EDITION

The *Ultimate Guides* from Cleis Press

The Ultimate Guide to Anal Sex for Women

SECOND EDITION

TRISTAN TAORMINO

ILLUSTRATED BY FISH

Published in the United States by Cleis Press Inc.,
P.O. Box 14697, San Francisco, California 94114.
Printed in the United States.
Cover design: Scott Idleman
Cover photograph: Donata Pizzi/Getty Images
Book design: Karen Quigg
Cleis Press logo art: Juana Alicia
Second Edition.
10 9 8 7

Library of Congress Cataloging-in-Publication Data

Taormino, Tristan, 1971-

    The ultimate guide to anal sex for women / by Tristan Taormino; illustrated by Fish.— 2nd ed.

       p. cm.

    Includes bibliographical references and index.

    ISBN 1-57344-221-6 (pbk.: alk. paper)

1. Sex instruction for women.   2. Anal sex.   3. Anus (Psychology)   I. Title.

    HQ46.T24 2006

      613.9'6—dc22   2005034243

Acknowledgments

There are so many people whom I'd like to thank for their contributions to this book.

To Felice Newman and Frédérique Delacoste, for their time, devotion, and gracious understanding. In 1997, they took a chance on a first-time author and a provocative subject, and I am forever grateful to them. Special thanks once again to Felice, to whom I dedicated the first edition, for going beyond the call of duty as an editor. Thank you to my copyeditor, Kevin Bentley.

So many people contributed to the success of the first edition, and some of them are Tom Bates, Rosana Francescato, Karen Green, Russ Kick, Robert Morgan, Chip Rowe, the folks at San Francisco Sex Information, Don Spargo, Jr., Howard Stern, and Don Weise.

To Joani Blank, Susie Bright, Patrick Califia, Debi Sundahl, Nina Hartley, Bert Herrman, Nan Kinney, Jack Morin, Carol Queen, Anne Semans, and Cathy Winks for their extraordinary, groundbreaking work. Without them, this book could not exist.

To Ray Cirino for his inspiration, Beth Tyler for her kick-ass website, the vixens at Vixen Creations for making my dream butt plug, and Shar Rednour and Jackie Strano for putting bend-over boyfriends on the map.

To Claire Cavanah, Rachel Venning, and everyone at Babeland for their support and the opportunity to work in such an important place.

To John Stagliano, Ernest Greene, Evil Angel, and the cast and crew of my video for bringing the book to life in an entertaining and educational way.

To the organizations, colleges, universities, and stores that have invited me to speak or teach about anal sex, and to the courageous people I have done anal demos on—including Barb, Carol, David, Frasier, George, Glenda, Janet, Jessica, Maggie, Marsha, Nancy, Nina, Paula, Sarafina, and Tracy. I learned so much from each of you.

To Thia "Fish" Jennings for her wit, her understanding, and her brilliant illustrations.

To Nancy Bereano of Firebrand Books, Joan Nestle, Greg Constante, Patrick Califia, and Sarah Miller for permission to reprint their work.

To Dr. Beth Brown for her medical expertise.

To Audrey, Barb, Betty, Carly, Clyde, David, Dylan, Greg, Helen, Ira, Julie, Kate, Kathy, Morgan, Nina, Tey, Toni, and Winston for their love and friendship.

To my mother and my late father for always supporting me no matter what.

To my partner Colten Tognazzini for teaching me about unconditional love, patience, and unlimited possibilities, and to our dogs—Reggie Love, Jordan, and Harley—who are my constant companions during research, reading, writing, and revisions.

Contents

Illustrations

Introduction:

Confessions of a Backdoor Betty...
Eight Years Later

Yes, I admit it—I love anal sex. The first time someone put a finger in my butt, I thought I'd died and gone to heaven. I think I almost went crazy from the pleasure. The sensations I experienced were so intense that I felt high from the experience, and I couldn't wait to do it again. The first time I put my finger in someone else's butt, the results were just as fabulous—I felt entrusted with my partner's deepest vulnerabilities, in awe of the ecstatic pleasure I could give. Then came more fingers, tongues, vibrators, small dildos, bigger dildos, butt plugs, cocks, bigger butt plugs, even an entire small hand. Each time I could take a little more and give a little more, I felt more sexually alive and powerful. As I incorporated anal eroticism into my sex life, my sex life became better and better. The sex got hotter, my partners more adventurous, my orgasms fierce and explosive. The physical sensations were undeniably some of the best I'd ever felt in my life. I confess too that beyond the deep body gratification, the naughtiness of it all really turned me on.

The opening paragraph of the introduction to the first edition of this book really says it all. It was my passion for anal sex that fueled my desire to write a book about it, and I'm pleased to say that my love for the subject, both intellectually and carnally, has only grown since the book was first published in late 1997.

When I sat down to research and write *The Ultimate Guide to Anal Sex for Women* in 1996 and 1997, there was very little information out there. At the time, there were books and articles on specific topics—solo sex, oral sex, vibrator sex, sex after fifty, fantasy role-playing sex, lesbian sex, phone sex, gay sex, Tantric sex, healing sex, cybersex, kinky sex—yet only one book devoted to the back door, *Anal Pleasure and Health* by Jack Morin. (I must continue to acknowledge and pay homage again to Jack Morin, who was so far ahead of his time, whom I still consider to be the king of anal pleasure, and whose work influenced me tremendously.) Other more general sex self-help manuals, of which there were plenty, dodged the topic of anal sex, devoted scant attention to it, or subtly dismissed it with misinformation that could scare readers away from exploring anal pleasure. Mentions of ass-fucking and ass loving—especially positive ones—in the media barely existed, with the exception of gay male erotica and both gay and straight porn videos.

I'm thrilled to say that in less than ten years a lot has changed. There is a new generation of sex books—titles like *Guide to Getting It On!* by Paul Joannides, *Nerve's Guide to Sex Etiquette for Ladies and Gentlemen* by Emma Taylor and Lorelei Sharkey, and *The Ultimate Guide to Cunnilingus* by Violet Blue—that include plenty of sex-positive info about anal pleasure. The butt is front and center in the *Bend Over Boyfriend* video series and makes appearances in new lesbian porn by S.I.R. Video. There's even *The Ultimate Guide to Anal Sex for Men!*

Ass sex is not only getting its fair shake in sex books and videos, it was the sole subject of former ballerina Toni Bentley's lauded memoir *The Surrender* and it turns up in mainstream media like *Redbook*, *The New York Times*, *The New Republic*, *Glamour*, and *Jane*. I spoke about anal sex on MSNBC, HBO, and the Discovery Channel, and it got plenty of airtime on *Sex and the City*.

Beginning with its auspicious debut on *The Howard Stern Show*, *The Ultimate Guide to Anal Sex for Women* took on a life of its own. I developed several workshops based on the book that I've taught to more than a thousand people around the world. I cannot count how many times I've illustrated anal penetration with my finger nestled in the pink puckered

A-hole of a men's masturbation device called the Fleshlight, while the rest of my digits wrapped around a bright green dildo, as I explained to a roomful of people how to get a dildo in someone's ass. In private and in public, I've put fingers, butt plugs, and dildos in the asses of friends, lovers, and complete strangers (the latter for demonstration purposes, of course). I made two videos based on the book and designed two butt plugs that were named after me. I've received thousands of letters from people, and answered hundreds of different questions. All this just goes to show that when you give people permission to discuss anal sex, they will. And I know from experience that lots of people want information about anal pleasure.

At lectures, workshops, hell, at cocktail parties, people from all walks of life approach me with inquiries about anal sex. Some follow up with: "Are you sick and tired of being asked about anal sex?" The answer remains the same: absolutely not. I welcome their questions—questions their doctors avoid, questions they can't ask their closest confidant, questions no high school health teacher I know would entertain—and I'm glad they had the courage to ask them.

Recently, at a class in New York, a beautiful blonde woman in a light blue sweater raised her hand and queried, "After the initial penetration of a guy's cock in your ass, when should it start to feel good?" "Honey, it should be feeling good all along, and if it's not, then something's wrong," I said. She went on to describe a first-time experience that was painful, something I know other women can relate to. "Was there warm-up, or did he just stick it in?" I asked. The latter, as I suspected. The guy sitting next to her even copped to being the owner of the (understandably) overzealous dick. I told them to make a pact: they will go slow, do plenty of warm-up, and, if it hurts at all, stop without any consequences—no frustration, no feeling guilty, on either side. "Once you're in," I told him, "don't go all the way. Hang back with just the head inside to allow her ass to get used to the feeling. Oh, and was there clitoral stimulation going on? Because you usually can't go wrong with some clit stimulation." They looked at each other, then back at me, smiling.

My job is never boring.

As a kid, I was taught by some pretty great, underappreciated public school teachers, and, although they weren't talking prostate glands and anal beads, they influenced the way I inform others about my favorite subject. I just put it all out there. Nothing is off limits: enemas, poop, hemorrhoids, why you shouldn't use Vaseline as lube or candles as sex toys. It's important not to shy away from the so-called embarrassing stuff and to just be honest. My goal is simple: debunk the myths, fight the taboos, explain the basics, and give people information and tools they can use. And do it in a way that's less boring lecture, more stand-up sass. I'm one of those teachers who wants to get my students so excited about the material that they beg for extra-credit assignments (hint: my butt toys need to be inventoried!). I challenge them ("Every man in this room should be fucked in the ass at least once before he dies!"), and I hope I inspire them. It feels good to know that I've contributed to improving someone's erotic awareness, and ultimately her sex life. Sometimes, I want to go home with my students (no, not like that…well, not with *all* of them anyway), peek into their bedroom for a night, and coach their anal pleasure session from plug to plow. But usually I must send them on their way with a reassuring nod and a tube of Astroglide Gel.

When I began work on this second edition, several friends asked me, "A second edition? Do you actually have *more* to say on the subject?" Well, as it turns out, I do. Through teaching anal sex classes, being asked questions I didn't know the answer to, having lots more anal sex (both in front of a roomful of students and in private), I have learned so much more. The publisher didn't just stick a new cover on the old book and call it "updated." Every single page has been revised; there are new chapters, new illustrations, new tips and techniques, new answers to new questions.

The title is still *The Ultimate Guide to Anal Sex for Women*, and it is written from a woman's perspective and geared toward all women, regardless of their sexual orientation. It's so important for women to have information and inspiration about our bodies and the pleasure they can bring us. That said, women aren't the only ones who bought the first edition, who attend my workshops, or who write to me, and I hope this edition can be equally useful for people of all genders. Although the book concentrates on the experiences of women, many of the guidelines and generalizations about anal sex apply to everyone.

Growing up in America, it is nearly impossible to escape the taboo about anal sexuality and all the myths surrounding it. From an early age, we are taught that our assholes are private, dirty, and shouldn't be touched in a sexual way. Whether we learn about the birds and the bees from popular books or in sex education class, the ass is rarely mentioned, unless to say it's behind our genitals. When anal sex is acknowledged as an erotic preference in sex research and popular advice columns, it is portrayed as a fantasy of straight men whose female partners endure pain in order to please them. There are rarely representations of women who enjoy anal sex with either men or women. Myths like these are based on fear more than fact, and often prevent people from voicing their anal desires and acting on those desires. The first chapter is a good place to begin exploring these myths more closely. If we challenge the deeply ingrained notions behind them and discover how they have affected our own attitudes about the ass and its erotic potential, we can begin to replace those myths with truths. In addition, you may find the facts useful for talking about anal sex with your partner.

In the second chapter, I provide a brief anatomy lesson, covering related muscles and body parts, and encourage you to get better acquainted with your ass. In chapter 3, I discuss some ways we can take care of ourselves emotionally and psychologically, covering topics like desire, communication, and fear. In addition, I explore some of the issues that may come up during anal sex with a partner, including fantasy, power dynamics, and trust. Chapters 4 and 5 cover basic preparation tips you should know about before beginning anal exploration, including hygiene, grooming, and enemas.

Safer sex practices are the subject of chapter 6, and there is a guide to lubricants in chapter 7. Sex toys are the focus of chapter 8, including anal beads, butt plugs, anal probes, dildos, vibrating and inflatable toys, and strap-ons. Plus, there are some hints about how to assess the safety of any other tool you're thinking of using for anal sex.

Chapters 9 through 11 cover the ins and outs of anal masturbation, analingus (also called rimming), and beginning and advanced anal penetration, including information on positions. Chapter 12 highlights specific issues and techniques for male anal pleasure. In chapters 13, 14, and 15, we move into more edgy territory, with BDSM, long-term butt plug wear, and anal fisting. Based on my work over the years, I've compiled a troubleshooting guide of some of the most common issues and problems people ask me about for chapter 16.

Chapter 17 is an important one for everyone; it covers general anal health, common anal ailments, as well as sexually transmitted diseases

(STDs)—their symptoms and treatments. The information about various diseases is written specifically as it relates to anal sexuality.

In each chapter, you'll see sidebars called Ask the Anal Advisor: these are questions from real people and my answers. Throughout the book, I have also included brief excerpts from erotic literature and quotes from popular books and magazines about anal pleasure. I hope these words will encourage you to enact your own anal fantasies and enjoy the full range of anal eroticism. At the end of the book, I have included a resource guide, with selected books, videos, websites, and other sources for people who want to learn more about anal pleasure.

I want this book to empower you with knowledge about your body and sexuality. I want you to have safe and pleasurable anal sex, alone or with your partners. And, while the cover touts this book as the "Ultimate Guide," I don't consider it the final word by any means. I hope it is just the beginning—the beginning of more discussion, more research, more investigation, and more exploration of the world of anal sexuality.

The moment I discovered anal eroticism and shared it with a lover was a huge turning point in my sex life. It still drives me crazy after all this time. I hope that you—beginner, fan, or expert—will use this book to help fulfill, improve, and enhance your explorations of anal pleasure.

Tristan Taormino
New York City
November 2005

12 Myths About Anal Sex

Myth #1: Anal sex is unnatural, wrong, and immoral.

TRUTH: Religion, medicine, science, government, education, media, and other important institutions dictate what is considered acceptable behavior (and what is considered deviant) in all areas of life, including sexuality. The anal sex taboo has been well established and reinforced by these institutions in order to maintain the status quo. For example, most sex education programs for students under eighteen do not include any mention of anal pleasure or anal sex. The majority of sex self-help books for adults include little or no information on the subject. When anal sex is represented in mainstream media (which is still infrequently), it is more often portrayed as negative, violent, or degrading than positive or pleasurable. Up until the 1960s, under sodomy laws, anal sex was a crime; in some states, it only applied to same-sex partners, while in others, it applied to everyone. As recently as this decade, it was still illegal for anyone to engage in anal sex in nine states in America. In the case of Lawrence v. Texas in 2003, the Supreme Court ruled that sodomy laws were unconstitutional.

*My best friend, Jane, called me
a few weeks ago.
"I beat you," she said.
"You beat me? You have a job, your
boyfriend went to Princeton, and you
live in a major city. I'm sporadically
employed in a town with, like, one
offramp, and my boyfriend went to
a minor Midwestern university and
thinks deodorant is bourgeois. The
only thing I have on you is that I'm
a bigger slut."
"That," she said, "is precisely how
I beat you."
"You had anal sex."
"Bingo."
My heart sank. "You must be
very pleased with yourself."
"Honey, you have no idea."*
—SARAH MILLER—

The good news is that history teaches us that sexual norms are constantly changing. There was a time when masturbation was thought to be unhealthy and sinful. In the 1970s, oral sex was considered out of the ordinary, even a little kinky. Today, masturbation and oral sex are considered a healthy part of a person's sex life. Today's taboo is tomorrow's norm.

Most of us have grown up learning something negative about our asses, so the myths that follow will sound familiar. The legacy of anal sex taboos continue to linger and inform how people perceive anal pleasure. New sexuality research, changes in sex education, and legal victories like Lawrence v. Texas will hopefully go a long way toward shifting public opinion.

Myth #2: Only sluts, perverts, and weirdos have anal sex.

TRUTH: The notion that anal sex is kinky, abnormal, or perverse is based on the assumption that one form of sexual expression—specifically, heterosexual penis-vagina intercourse—is natural, normal, and conventional. All other activities, including manual stimulation, oral sex, and sex toys, are considered abnormal. From the perky girl next door to the daring dominatrix in the dungeon, people of every age, gender, sexual orientation, socio-economic class, race, religion, occupation, and ability practice and enjoy anal sex.

Myth #3: The ass is exit only, it's not an erogenous zone.

TRUTH: It's true that the anus and rectum are parts of our body's efficient waste management system. But, in addition, the ass is full of sensitive, responsive nerve endings, and the stimulation of these nerve endings can be intensely pleasurable—and orgasmic—for both men and women. When we get turned on, and our pussies get wet, our cocks and clits erect, our asses aren't left out. They too become engorged, aroused, and extra sensitive. Through anal penetration, women can experience indirect G-spot stimulation and men get direct prostate stimulation.

ASK THE ANAL ADVISOR: *Am I Normal?*

Q: *I've been married over fifteen years and my husband has suggested anal sex a couple of times, and he even rubbed around my butt a few times, but as a "good girl," I never wanted to go further. That changed on my husband's fortieth birthday. I offered him my butt to do as he wished and I have to admit I really, really liked it (even though it was a bit sore the next morning). That was three years ago. I never thought that I would enjoy anal sex as much as I do. Now, I often think that I prefer anal sex, and most of our intercourse includes some sort of anal play. Is it normal to like anal sex as much or better than vaginal sex? Am I an anal addict?*

A: And what a great birthday present you gave your husband! To answer your question simply and directly, there is really no such thing as "normal." Mainstream culture and media would have us believe that heterosexual cock-in-pussy intercourse is the most common activity and therefore normal, but we all know that is bull. The truth is that we like what we like. Whether it's the smack of a riding crop on your butt, an enthusiastic toe-sucking, or anal play, if it turns you and your partner on, then go for it! For some women, anal penetration may feel as good as or better than vaginal penetration; lots of people tell me that anal play produces more intense orgasms. Plus, adding clitoral stimulation to backdoor banging or creating an angle for indirect G-spot stimulation can all help increase the pleasure of anal penetration. It sounds like you really enjoy anal sex with your husband; ignore those voices in your head which may be calling you deviant or weird, and just keep doing what you're doing.

Myth #4: Anal sex is dirty and messy.

TRUTH: In general, Americans have an obsession with hygiene and cleanliness, so this myth plays into our fears of being dirty. We imagine our asses to be a lot filthier than they actually are. Feces are stored in the colon and pass through the rectum and out the anus during a bowel movement. If you're a healthy person with regular bowel movements, than only a small amount of fecal matter will be present in the anal canal and rectum. As long as you practice standard hygiene, anal sex is no more messy than any other kind of sex. If you have a bowel movement and take a shower or bath before sex to clean the anal area, no other extraordinary measures are needed. Some people like to have an enema before anal sex, but that is not necessary.

Myth #5: Only gay men have anal sex.

TRUTH: People of all genders and sexual orientations have anal sex. While it's true that many gay men do have anal sex, the actual statistics reveal a much smaller percentage than is widely believed: 50–60 percent have tried it and fewer than 30 percent have it regularly. Fellatio is a much more common practice among gay men.[1] The idea that *all* gay men and *only* gay men have anal sex—one that the Religious Right would like us to believe—is simply not supported. Furthermore, there is no evidence that any single group defined by sexual orientation has a great deal more anal sex than any other group. In fact, depending on which survey you cite, from 20 to 45 percent of women have anal sex.[2]

Myth #6: Straight men who like anal sex are really gay.

TRUTH: Men who like anal sex (whether they are on the giving or receiving end) like it because it feels good. Their desire for buttfucking has nothing to do with their sexual orientation, and this myth is fueled by homophobia. Heterosexual men who like anal sex are not repressing homosexual desires or tendencies. Their desire for a particular sexual activity does not rely on or "cancel out" their sexual preference in a partner. According to research, more gay men regularly practice fellatio than anal sex, and as my friend Audrey says, "How come no one ever asks: If a straight guy likes blow jobs, does that mean he's really gay?"

Ask the Anal Advisor: *Am I Gay?*

Q: *I'm a guy, I like women, and I've never been attracted in any way to men. I want to try anal sex (with me on the receiving end) with dildos and even a strap-on. Does this mean I am gay?*

A: The idea that men who like getting it up the butt are gay is absolutely a myth, one fueled by our society's homophobia and misconceptions about anal pleasure. Plenty of heterosexual men enjoy receiving anal pleasure, whether with tongues, fingers, or toys. As I've said before, anal sex can be an incredibly powerful experience, but it's not powerful enough to change your sexual orientation! I think that men who enjoy strap-on action especially have anxiety because of the implication that they are getting fucked by a cock, whether it's silicone or not. The truth is that it feels good, and when you turn around, you want a woman on the other end of that cock.

Myth #7: Anal sex hurts.

TRUTH: Anal sex should not hurt—not even a little. If it hurts, you're doing something wrong. Pain is your body's way of saying, "This is not working for me right now," and we must listen to our bodies. If you ignore your body's warnings and continue, then you can hurt yourself. The experience may make you and your anus more tense the next time you try anal penetration. Your body remembers everything, so don't try to fool it. You don't have to "work through the pain" to get to the pleasure. That's what you do at the gym, not during anal sex. With desire, relaxation, communication, and lots of lubrication, anal sex can be not only pain-free but arousing and orgasmic.

Myth #8: Women don't like anal sex.

TRUTH: This is a particularly insidious myth about heterosexual women. Often, when we do hear about women having anal sex, the story goes something like this: The long-term boyfriend begged and begged, and finally his girlfriend gave in to his demands. Her boyfriend had a great time, but she did it just to please him and didn't enjoy herself one bit.

"Buttfucking is seen as the ultimate male sexual fantasy. We, as a culture, don't understand how much women can like taking it up the ass."
— SUSAN CRAIN BAKOS—

We never hear stories about women who crave and enjoy anal play, women who initiate anal sex, or women who are more than happy to knock on their boyfriends' back door. Women all over the world write to me, come to my workshops, buy my books and videos, and they're just a small percentage of women everywhere who love anal sex.

Myth #9: Anal sex is dangerous and unhealthy.

TRUTH: Because anal and rectal tissue is so delicate, you can hurt yourself or someone else if you don't exercise all the precautions I discuss in this book. However, if you go slow, use plenty of lube, and listen to your body, anal sex is just as safe as any other kind of penetration. In fact, anal sex can make your butt better than it was before. The more you practice controlling and relaxing your sphincter muscles, the more you are exercising and toning them (just like any other muscle) as well as increasing blood flow to the area, all of which can improve the health of your ass.

Myth #10: If you have lots of anal sex, you'll end up in adult diapers.

TRUTH: When done properly, frequent penetration will not lead to a gaping asshole, loose sphincter muscles, or a loss of control over bowel movements. During anal penetration, you're not stretching or tearing the sphincter muscles; you are relaxing them to allow for comfortable penetration. With regular anal sex, you can get in touch with your sphincters and you may find that you actually have better bowel control than you did before.

Myth #11: Anal sex is the easiest way to get AIDS.

TRUTH: During anal penetration, you can develop minute tears in the delicate rectal tissue, which give any virus (including HIV) a direct route into the bloodstream. You can contract any sexually-transmitted disease, including HIV, from unprotected anal intercourse with an infected partner. Other forms of anal pleasure without safer sex barriers, including oral-anal contact, manual penetration, or sharing sex toys, can also be risky. However, anal sex does not *automatically* lead to AIDS. Anal sex practiced with common sense, safer sex, or an HIV-negative partner can be as safe as other sexual practices. (Read more about safer sex in Chapter 6 and STDs and HIV in Chapter 17.)

Myth #12: Anal sex is naughty.

TRUTH: Well, this is actually a myth *and* a truth. Of course, anal sex doesn't make you a bad person. However, for those of you who are turned on by the idea that anal sex is taboo, deviant, and naughty, don't let me ruin your party. Lots of people actually like the fact that anal sex is naughty, and they may incorporate that into their anal play. The "naughtiness factor" is part of the turn-on.

Replacing Myths with Truths

What did you learn about anal sex during your childhood, your teens, your adulthood? We all have some "negative cultural baggage" associated with our butts. We may laugh it off, but the most damaging thing about these myths, which are pervasive in our society, is that they prevent people from considering anal pleasure or from acting on their anal desires. If you have fears and anxieties about anal pleasure, you need to voice them, to yourself and to your partner. By acknowledging and discussing the myths that affect us in a safe environment, we can begin to see the truths behind the myths. Only then can we begin to see anal sex for what it really can be—safe, fun, and pleasurable.

NOTES

1. Jack Morin, *Anal Pleasure and Health* (San Francisco: Yes/Down There Press, 1986), 9-12, and June M. Reinisch with Ruth Beasley, *The Kinsey Institute New Report on Sex* (New York: St. Martin's Press, 1990), 137.

2. Elliot Leland and Cynthia Brantley, *Sex on Campus: The Naked Truth About the Real Sex Lives of College Students* (New York: Random House, 1997); Robert T. Michael et al., *Sex in America: A Definitive Survey* (New York: Little, Brown and Co., 1994); Samuel S. Janus and Cynthia L. Janus, *The Janus Report on Sexual Behavior* (New York: John Wiley & Sons, 1993); Reinisch and Beasley, *The Kinsey Institute New Report on Sex*; Morin, *Anal Pleasure and Health*.

QUOTES AND SIDEBARS

Sarah Miller, "The Slut Within," *Details* (The Sex Issue), May 1997, 77. © by Sarah Miller, reprinted with permission of the author.

Susan Crain Bakos, *Kink: The Hidden Sex Lives of Americans* (New York: St. Martin's Press, 1995), 7.

2

Our Asses, Ourselves:
Anal Anatomy

Although anatomy is part of science and medicine, the study of anatomy is less objective than one might think. There are a variety of differing interpretations and opinions about the internal structure of our bodies—especially the nuances and complexities of our sexual anatomy. This is certainly true for anorectal anatomy—which is nearly identical in men and women, except that men have a prostate gland. The discussion of anatomy and the anatomical illustrations in this book are based on my interpretations of several sources, including medical textbooks, sex manuals, and conversations with sex educators.[1]

The Anus

The anus is the external opening of the anal canal. It can be one of our most sensual erogenous zones, but it is one too often feared, forgotten, and left unexplored. It is comprised of folds of soft tissue that give it a wrinkled or puckered appearance. The area around the opening is full of hair follicles; the hair may be fine and light, coarse and dark, or somewhere in between. Everyone has hair surrounding the anus. Rich in blood vessels and nerve endings, the tissue of the anus is incredibly sensitive and responsive to touch and stimulation. Contrary to cultural mythology, with regular bathing and good personal hygiene, the anus is generally clean.

The Anal Sphincters and PC Muscles

Two muscles—the anal sphincters—surround the anal opening (see illustrations 1 and 2). The external sphincter is closest to the opening. With patience and practice, you can voluntarily control the external sphincter, making it tense or relax. Imagine that you are holding something in your ass or expelling something. As you suck in and tense up or push down and release, you are exercising your external sphincter muscles. The internal sphincter is controlled by the autonomic nervous system, which controls involuntary bodily functions like your breathing rate. This muscle ordinarily reacts reflexively; for example, when you are ready to have a bowel movement, the internal sphincter relaxes, allowing feces to move from the rectum to the anal canal and out the anus. Because the external and the internal sphincters overlap, they often work together. Think of the sphincter muscles as the gatekeepers to your ass. If they are relaxed, ready, aroused,

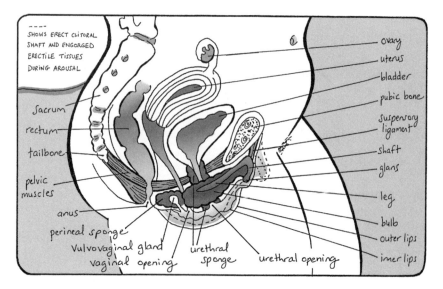

Illustration 1: Female Anatomy

and content, anal penetration will be comfortable and feel good. If they are tense, tight, or not warmed up, anal penetration will be uncomfortable, painful, or downright impossible.

Ask the Anal Advisor: *Changing Color*

Q: *Is there any way of making my anus pinker or lighter in color? Mine is dark and I hate it. Any suggestions?*

A: Several people have written to me asking me about skin bleaching in the anal area. First, let me assure you that the way your ass looks now is perfectly normal; in most people, the puckered flesh of the anus is naturally a few shades darker—or a slightly different color—than the rest of their skin. For some people, the contrast is more extreme than others.

Skin bleaching products are used to suppress pigmentation in order to lighten the skin; the most common products contain hydroquinone, kojic acid, or mandelic acid. There are two companies I know of that sell a product called anal bleaching cream, which they claim lightens the skin around the anus. Pink Cheeks Salon in Southern California produces and sells its own cream which contains 4 percent hydroquinone; ShopinPrivate.com sells a cream normally marketed for lightening freckles, age spots, and skin discoloration that contains 2 percent hydroquinone. Neither is approved by the FDA specifically for the bleaching of the anal area, although products with similar ingredients are approved for skin lightening. Consult a dermatologist or other physician before using any product on your ass.

As for making it more pink, well that's a little trickier. The pinkest holes I've ever seen are those that have been stroked, licked, and/or fucked until they couldn't help but blush with contentment (lots of blood rushing to the area helps, too). I support people modifying their bodies in whatever ways they wish in order to feel better about themselves, and so I offer you the information you requested; however, I would also like you to consider why you "hate" the way your ass looks, and what might be at the root of that particular body issue for you. Coming to terms with your negative feelings about your butt and learning to accept and love your body as it is will be a lot less painful and expensive and, in the end, seems like the "rosier" option.

Other surrounding muscles also contribute to sensations in the anal area. The perineal muscles support the area between the anus and the genitals. In this muscle group are the pubococcygeus muscles (PC muscles), which support the pelvis from the pubic bone to the tailbone. For both men and women, these muscles contract during sexual arousal and climax; specifically, they usually contract randomly when you are aroused and rhythmically during orgasm.

The more attention you pay to your sphincter muscles, the easier it will be to begin to relax them. Because the two muscles work in tandem, you can encourage the internal sphincter to relax by relaxing the external sphincter. Many people have found that by exercising and strengthening their PC muscles they can have more control of their sphincter muscles. PC muscle exercises will help you get in tune with the feelings in your pelvic area, increasing your sensitivity and responsiveness. The exercises will also tone the pelvic muscles, making them more flexible and more receptive to pleasurable sensations; plus, when you exercise the PC muscles, other muscles in the area are also exercised and strengthened. (For exercise examples, see Exercising Your PC Muscles below.)

Women and men who regularly exercise their PC and pelvic muscles report some very positive benefits: heightened pelvic sensations and greater anal sensitivity; increased pleasure during clitoral stimulation, and during vaginal and anal penetration; more control over orgasms; and better, more intense orgasms. As with any exercise regimen, this should be performed daily for best results. If your muscles seem tired at first, don't worry—that's normal. The harder the exercises are for you, the less toned your PC muscles are, and the more you need a workout. Use your common sense, and don't overdo it to begin with. If you experience any pain while doing them, see a doctor.

Unconscious internal sphincter, conscious external sphincter, only centimeters apart. Where else is one's unconscious and conscious mind so intimately connected, so readily regulated, so easily probed? It is a psychological playground of the most intriguing potential.
—TONI BENTLEY—

Exercising Your PC Muscles

Some of the following exercises are called Kegel exercises, named for the physician who first popularized the theory of exercising PC muscles; others are those recommended by health care professionals.[2] You can do the exercises lying down, sitting, or standing. You can also do them during masturbation or foreplay; you'll get a work out in addition to increasing blood flow to the area and upping your arousal.

FINDING THEM: In order to locate your PC muscles, pretend that you are trying to stop peeing (or while you are peeing, you can actually stop the flow of urine). The muscles you contract to stop the flow are your PC muscles. If you put your finger on your perineum—the area between your vagina and your anus—while you do this exercise, you can feel the contractions.

NICE AND EASY: Take a deep breath and while you inhale, contract the muscles and hold the contraction for a few seconds. Then exhale and relax the muscles. This combination of inhale/contract and exhale/relax is what your body does naturally. You can do about a hundred repetitions per day.

QUICK AND CLEAN: Take a deep breath and this time while you inhale, tighten and release the muscles repeatedly (about ten times), then exhale and relax. Try to do these contractions as quickly as you can. Twenty to fifty sets a day is recommended.

SUCK IT IN: For this exercise, inhale and pretend you are sucking water inside your vagina and anus. Then exhale and bear down, pushing out that imaginary water. You will exercise your pelvic muscles and your stomach muscles. For best results, do ten to thirty each day.

SHAKE IT GIRL: Renowned anal health expert Jack Morin recommends moving your body while you do your pelvic exercises: "I suggest combining the Kegel exercises with lots of free movement in a variety of settings. The positive effects of this movement will be limited, however, if you hold your pelvis rigid while moving the rest of your body. In fact, habitual, chronic, pelvic 'holding on' is one major reason why so many people need Kegel exercises. Holding the pelvis requires muscular tension which restricts movement. Restricted movement allows muscles to deteriorate."[3] Try combining the exercises with walking, running, dancing, or simulating a hula-hoop motion.

The Anal Canal and the Rectum

Just inside the anus is the anal canal. The anal canal is about one to two inches long and leads into the rectum. The same soft tissue that makes up the anus comprises the anal canal, so it is very sensitive to touch and stimulation. The walls of the anal canal are comprised of tissue that, like that of the clitoris and penis, becomes engorged from increased blood flow during arousal. When the sphincter muscles are relaxed, the anal canal will expand during arousal, although it will still feel "tighter" than the rectum because of the sphincter muscles.

Beyond the anal canal is the rectum, which is eight to nine inches long; the rectum is made up of loose folds of soft, smooth tissue. It is wider than the anal canal and can expand more than the anal canal when you are aroused. Unlike the vagina, the rectum is not a straight tube, but has

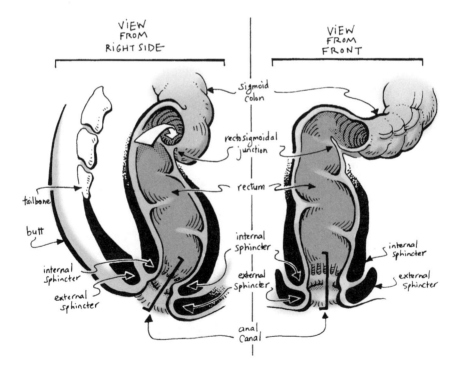

Illustration 2: Anorectal Anatomy

a subtle curve to it. The lower part of the rectum curves toward your navel. After a few inches, the rectum curves back toward your spine, then toward your navel again. The rectum and colon both curve laterally (from side to side) as well; whether to the right or the left will vary from person to person. These curves are part of the reason that anal penetration should be slow and gentle, especially at first. Each person's rectum and its curves are unique, and it is best to feel your way inside the rectum slowly, following its curves, rather than jamming anything straight inside. Just as the vagina is most sensitive at its opening, the anal opening and anal canal are more sensitive then the rectum.

A person's butt is as unique as a fingerprint.
—BERT HERRMAN—

The G-spot

Men's and women's anal anatomy is very similar with one important difference: women have a G-spot and men have a prostate gland, both of which can be stimulated during anal penetration. Named in honor of the German gynecologist Ernest Grafenberg who was the first to write about this sensitive spot in the 1950s, the G-spot is also known as the urethral sponge.[4] The G-spot is located behind the pubic bone; it surrounds a portion of a woman's urethra, and can be felt through the front wall of the vagina, about an inch to two inches inside the vaginal opening. It's much easier to find the G-spot when a woman is aroused, because during arousal, the sponge will swell and become more pronounced. If you slip a finger inside the vagina and curve toward the front of the body, you'll locate the G-spot, which will feel spongy, a distinctly different texture than the smooth tissue around it. For many, but not all women, stimulation of the G-spot is very pleasurable and may lead to orgasm. Most women who like G-spot stimulation prefer firm, deliberate pressure and stimulation rather than a light touch. The urethral sponge contains paraurethral glands and ducts that fill with fluid; some women are able to ejaculate this fluid. This is known as female ejaculation or vaginal ejaculation.

So what's the G-spot got to do with anal pleasure for women? During anal penetration, especially in certain positions, many women can experience indirect G-spot stimulation. A thin membrane is all that separates the vaginal cavity from the rectal cavity, and if pressure is applied at the right angle during anal penetration, the G-spot can be stimulated. In fact, plenty of women can have what they describe as a "G-spot orgasm" (the same orgasm they have from direct G-spot stimulation) during anal penetration, and some can ejaculate from anal penetration alone. Because it develops from the same embryologic tissue as the male prostate gland and produces fluid similar to prostatic fluid, the G-spot is often called the "female prostate."

The Prostate

The prostate is a gland that surrounds part of a man's urethra; it's behind the pubic bone, below the bladder, and above the base of the penis. A mass of muscle, glands, and connective tissue, the prostate is about the size and shape of a walnut; it produces ejaculatory fluid that combines with sperm and fluid from the seminal vesicles to create male ejaculate.

Men can experience direct prostate stimulation when they are anally penetrated. You can find the prostate two to three inches into the ass and toward the front of the body. Like the G-spot, it's easiest to find when a guy is turned on. As he becomes aroused, the prostate gland fills with fluid, swells, and becomes more prominent. Prostate stimulation can be a big

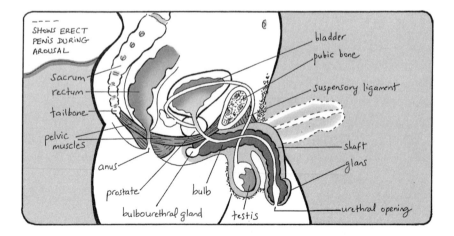

Illustration 3: Male Anatomy

source of pleasure for men; it can enhance genital stimulation as well as lead to orgasm. Many men can have an orgasm without ejaculation or ejaculate only prostatic fluid as a result of prostate stimulation. For more information on prostate stimulation, see chapter 12.

NOTES

1. Jack Morin, *Anal Pleasure and Health*; Cathy Winks and Anne Semans, *The New Good Vibrations Guide to Sex* (San Francisco: Cleis Press, 1997); Roselyn Payne Epps and Susan Cobb Stewart, eds., *The American Medical Women's Association Guide to Sexuality* (New York: Dell Books, 1996); James H. Grendell, M.D., Kenneth R. McQuaid, M.D., and Scott L. Friedman, M.D., eds., *Current Diagnosis and Treatment in Gastroenterology* (New York: Simon & Schuster, 1996); and San Francisco sex educator Robert Morgan, personal conversations.

2. These exercises are recommended in *Anal Pleasure and Health,* by Jack Morin, and *The Complete Guide to Safer Sex from the Institute for Advanced Study of Human Sexuality,* edited by Ted McIlvenna (Fort Lee, NJ: Barricade Books, 1992).

3. Morin, *Anal Pleasure,* 59.

4. Beverly Whipple, John D. Perry, and Alice Khan Ladas, *The G Spot: And Other Discoveries About Human Sexuality* (New York: Owl Books, 2005).

QUOTES AND SIDEBARS

Toni Bentley, *The Surrender: An Erotic Memoir* (New York: ReganBooks, 2004), 87.

Bert Herrman, *Trust: The Hand Book (A Guide to the Sensual and Spiritual Art of Handballing)* (San Francisco: Alamo Square Press, 1991), 45.

3

Beyond Our Bodies:
Emotional and Psychological Aspects of Anal Eroticism

Our emotional, psychological, and spiritual well-being play a major role in our erotic lives, and our experiences of anal sexuality are no exception. Anal play can be exceptionally psychologically-charged for some of us because of our own emotional issues or negative ideas associated with the ass. Listen to your heart, trust your instincts, and, above all, communicate with your partner.

Desire

There really is no faking it in anal sex. Your body, mind, and psyche all must be in agreement that you want to have anal sex. Don't have anal sex because you think it's what your partner wants. Or because your partner is pressuring you to do it. Or because you're afraid that you won't be a desirable lover if you don't do it. Take responsibility for your erotic likes and dislikes—figure out what they are and then communicate them to your partner. If you aren't wholeheartedly gung ho about getting your ass fucked or you're harboring some unresolved issues, those emotional and psychological feelings will absolutely have an impact on your physical experience. Desire is a key ingredient to hot, satisfying anal sex, and if it's missing, you can experience tension, discomfort, and pain. If you try it and don't like it, then that's okay; anal sex just isn't for you, and you should respect your own desires.

The most important thing, the single most important thing when you're talking about wanting to progress forward with any kind of anal erotic play is desire. You must, must do this because you want to do it... Of all the parts of your body, nothing knows a liar like your anus. So if your mind is saying "Yes! Yes!" and your heart is saying "No! No!" your anus will always listen to your heart.
— NINA HARTLEY —

Talking About It

Communication is a key component before, during, and after anal sex. Communication about sex is specific to the individuals involved, so there's no one rule that will work for everyone. No matter how you approach it, it's a good idea to talk to your partner about this in a nonsexual setting, rather than *right* before you're about to delve into anal erotic play. Depending on how your partner reacts, it could bring things to a screeching halt, which no one wants. You can go about it in a number of different ways, and how you do it should depend on your style and your partner's comfort level. You may want to test the waters in a playful, indirect way. Try a statement that will let you see what your partner thinks about the subject in general, like, "I saw something in this magazine about anal sex, what do you think about it?" This is a safe way to approach it if you're not sure how your partner may react. Saying, "I want to do *this* to *you*. *Now*," can put pressure on a person to respond immediately or may make someone feel more intimidated or threatened. If you and your partner are direct with each other and talk openly about sex, then, by all means, be direct. But if you're hesitant, give your partner time to react; tell him or her you don't need a response right away. It's important that you make your request as pressure-free as possible, and give her the opportunity to voice her concerns, if she has any.

No lover is able to look into your eyes and figure out how you want to get fucked in the ass.
—SUSIE BRIGHT—

ASK THE ANAL ADVISOR: *Hesitant Partner*

Q: *I have been with my girlfriend for six years, going on seven. The sex is really amazing, but something is missing: anal. I love to eat her pussy a lot. The taste of her and just being down there can make me come. For the past year, when we sixty-nine, as I lick her pussy, I have been playing with her ass, and she moans louder when I do that. One time, my whole thumb was in her ass and she loved it. But when we talk about it, she seems hesitant. When I go down on her, I tend to give her a small rim job or, when we are in the missionary position and I swivel her left leg over so her ass is exposed, I play with her ass. She gets into it, and then stops. I'm very confused. I think she loves it, but I don't know.*

A: It sounds to me like you two need to have a conversation about anal pleasure. According to your account, your girlfriend isn't opposed to it, though it seems that you want to go further than she is comfortable going. It may be that rimming and penetration with a finger feel great, and she has no desire to do any more. But the fact that you're getting mixed signals means she may have some unexplored issues that prevent her from fully enjoying the anal play you already do and stop her from further exploration. Be open, compassionate, and nonjudgmental when you approach her. Ask her if she has fears or misgivings about anal pleasure; she may have concerns about hygiene, safer sex, penetration, and other common issues associated with butt sex. Talk through these issues, and see if you can get to the bottom of her feelings.

Fear

People can have a lot of fears and negative feelings about anal eroticism. In some cases, a partner may be hesitant about knockin' on the back door because she has certain misconceptions about buttfucking—that it's dirty, painful, or only for a man's pleasure. They seem irrational on the page, but these are very real fears in people's minds that may prevent them from even considering it. It is important to realize that most of us are made aware of the anal taboo starting in childhood and therefore we are all affected in some way by it.

While most of these fears have their roots in myths and misconceptions about anal sex, it is important to respect and validate your partner when she or he shares her or his feelings. Have an honest talk with your partner about fears you both have, and review chapter 1 and its discussion of myths, dispelling the misinformation and replacing it with correct information: anal sex doesn't have to be a big mess; if you do it right, it won't hurt; and women can get off on it in plenty of ways. Reassure each other that either one of you can stop the activity at any time and be fully supported by the other one. Set concrete ground rules and boundaries about what is okay and what isn't; as experiences progress, the boundaries can change if needed. Each person needs to know that she or he will be safe from both pain and disease during anal sex and that there is mutual trust and respect.

Some people's fears may be about anal sex being difficult, uncomfortable, painful, or impossible to enjoy. Women especially often veto anal sex because of a negative experience in the past. If a past partner tried to go from zero to sixty in five seconds by sticking his dick in your ass without warm-up, lube, or communication, then chances are it hurt a lot and you never want to do it again. Bad sexual experiences are difficult to overcome: who'd want to repeat something awful? Your partner needs to reassure you: this time, with him, it will be different. He'll take his time, use plenty of lube, and work your ass up to his cock. You will be in control of the pace, and he'll stop if you say so.

On the flip side, the partner who'll be doing the penetrating can also have fears. You may be afraid that you'll hurt your partner, you won't do it right, or you won't like it. The important thing is that you get everything out on the table before you begin your anal adventure.

Having an open, honest discussion can help illuminate what each person wants from the experience and why, so both people are less likely to make incorrect assumptions about the other person's desires and expectations. You can ask each other: What do you want? What do you expect? What are your needs? Here are some examples of what a receptive partner might say:

I'm afraid it will feel okay, but I'll never want to do it again.

I want to work my way up to one finger, then stop.

I'd like licking and touching, but no penetration.

I want to be able to have the small dildo in my butt.

We've done fingers a dozen times, tonight I want your cock.

I want everything to feel safe.

What have your previous experiences been with anal eroticism? Share them, discuss them. Why do you want to explore anal sensuality? Insertive partners should share as much as receivers:

I want to explore something new with you.

I'm curious about what it feels like.

I've done it before and want to do it again.

It's something special and intimate that I want to share with you.

I saw it in a porn movie, it turned me on, and I want to try it.

It's always been a fantasy of mine.

Fantasies

Fantasies can be incredibly powerful forces in our lives, erotic and otherwise. Many people fantasize about erotic activities like anal sex but are afraid to vocalize their desires. Sharing our sexual fantasies with a partner can deepen a sexual relationship and help us communicate our needs and desires.

Some people have very specific fantasies associated with anal play. Maybe you want to dominate your partner as you fuck his or her ass. Or you have a fantasy of being fucked in the ass against your will. Perhaps you want to play out a doctor-patient scenario, get your temperature taken with a rectal thermometer, and take it from there. Some men like to take on a female persona, willingly or as "forced feminization" when they get fucked in the ass. With anal play fantasies, the possibilities are endless.

It is equally important to distinguish our fantasies from our realities. If your favorite masturbatory fantasy involves someone ramming your butt repeatedly with a giant silicone dick that makes you come every time, don't be surprised if you don't get the same result when you try it out. There are some fantasies that we can share and help bring to life, others we have to tweak slightly based on what's realistic and our own boundaries, and others that should probably remain fantasies. Have realistic expectations for yourself and know the limits of your own body. One finger in your ass and a whisper in your ear about that big dick might just do the trick.

Trust and Power

Anal sex can be very charged, intense, and emotional. There are power dynamics in all sexual interactions, but they can be especially magnified during anal sex because it is such a forbidden act and because of the physical delicacy of the anus and rectum. Think about it: you're giving a delicate part of your body over to another person. That can raise deep issues of power and trust.

It's important for partners to be able to discuss their feelings openly, feel safe, and trust one another. The person receiving anal penetration can feel especially vulnerable, both physically and emotionally, and the partner giving anal pleasure must respect the receiver's wishes, needs, and limits. The giver may fear that she or he will hurt the receiving partner and needs to be reassured that everything's okay. Again, communication and ground rules can help alleviate tension and reassure both people that it will be a pain-free, safe experience.

Because of the trust involved, it's important for both partners to be completely present. Too often, people who attend my workshops or write to me say, "I can only have anal sex if I've had five drinks." I'm not going to deny that people combine alcohol and drugs and pleasurable anal sex. Ultimately, alcohol and drugs of any kind alter your awareness of your body, an awareness you absolutely must have to enjoy anal sex. Anal sex requires of both partners patience, skill, good communication, and coordination. The insertive partner needs to be keenly aware, intuitive, and able to read her or his partner's body language and nonverbal cues. The receiver needs to be in touch with his or her body to know what feels good and what doesn't—especially if he or she is a novice. People are more likely to ignore their anal boundaries—both physical and mental—if their judgment is impaired by alcohol and drugs. I believe that with proper relaxation, communication, trust, and desire, people can experience pleasurable anal intercourse without any "help" from alcohol or drugs. The intimacy and ecstasy of anal pleasure can sometimes be overwhelming, but it can also be very special and extremely satisfying, especially if both partners are fully present and connected.

QUOTES

Nina Hartley, *Nina Hartley's Guide to Anal Sex* (Adam and Eve Productions, 1994).

Susie Bright, "Ass Forward" in *Susie Sexpert's Lesbian Sex World* (San Francisco: Cleis Press, 1990), 34.

Preparing the Ass
for Pleasure

The best thing you can do to make anal sex more comfortable and clean is to clear the runway: have a bowel movement beforehand. Feces are stored in the colon, and only move into the rectum just before a bowel movement. If you feel the urge to go and listen to it, feces pass through the rectum and out of the body. (If you cannot or do not go to the bathroom at that moment and instead hold it in, feces will remain in the rectum until you do go.)

If you are in good general health and have well-formed bowel movements, then the rectum and anus will be generally free of fecal matter after you go. However, if your poop isn't perfect—due to poor diet, stress, constipation, diarrhea, or other gastrointestinal problems—there may be more fecal matter present in the rectum. In that case, you may want to have an enema before anal sex. (For more on enemas, read chapter 5.)

Even the healthiest rectums may contain trace amount of fecal matter, so it's important to be realistic about your expectations for anal play. As adult film star Chloe says, "Get over your fear of shit!"[1] She's right. Feces pass through your ass on a regular basis, so expecting to never encounter some during anal play is unrealistic. I am not saying you need to love or even like contact with feces, but the more anal play you engage in, the more likely it will happen. You might as well just smile, clean up, and move on.

Hygiene

Before sex, take a shower or a bath and clean your genitals. I recommend that people use castile soap—a very mild soap made from coconut, hemp, or olive oils, or a combination of oils—to clean their private parts. Most bar soaps, liquid antibacterial soaps, and body washes contain harsh ingredients like dyes and fragrances that can irritate sensitive skin and mucous membranes. While bathing, you may want to stick a soapy finger up your ass to gently clean out the anal canal. Make sure you rinse your ass well afterward. If, for whatever reason, you can't bathe, you can use a wet washcloth or a baby wipe to clean the anal area. In fact, I like to have a box of baby wipes nearby during an anal play session. Baby wipes are made for the genital area and much less harsh than other wipes, like Wet Ones. I like the baby wipes that are unscented and alcohol-free because the "baby" smell isn't erotic for me, and the alcohol-free wipes tend to be gentler on my delicate parts. They are great for catching lube drips and cleaning up unexpected messes.

Manicured Nails

The tissue of the anus, anal canal, and rectum is very delicate, much more delicate than the tissue of the vagina. If you're planning to use your fingers to stimulate your ass or your partner's, make sure your nails are short and filed smooth. Check for torn cuticles, or jagged or sharp edges, which can be felt inside the sensitive ass. Short, smooth nails will help prevent small tears in the anal tissue, which can cause irritation and discomfort during or after anal play. If you're not sure about your nails, you may choose to wear a latex or latex-alternative glove. Gloves aren't just a safer sex barrier: they transform your hand into a smooth, seamless tool for comfortable stimulation and penetration. For more about gloves, see chapter 6.

Ask the Anal Advisor: *Long Fingernails*

Q: *My boyfriend seems to like my finger up his butt when I suck his cock. I am worried, however, that I might hurt or scratch him because I have nice long fingernails, and I hate to cut them. Any advice?*

A: So much pleasure awaits both of you, but you're smart to be concerned about your nails. The sensitive anus and rectum require gentle handling. Don't despair—you can keep your long nails and still give him what he wants. First, you need to invest in some disposable latex or nonlatex gloves. To protect you partner and prevent a tear in the glove, stuff a cotton ball in each fingertip. Or you can wrap your nails in gauze before slipping on a glove. One woman recently told me she's found a finger bandage which she puts on underneath a latex glove. Whichever option you choose, make sure you use plenty of lube on your glove.

Shaving and Waxing

I love to shave my ass in addition to shaving my pussy. I am proud to say that I can shave my ass without a mirror. I am so familiar with every millimeter of my ass that I can just feel my way around all the puckered flesh and tiny, sensitive folds. I love the way my ass (and my pussy) feels when it's been freshly shaved—smooth and soft and new. I love the potential danger of doing it, and the results of a job well done. I love the thought of someone pulling down my panties, bending me over, and thinking, *What a nicely shaved asshole she has.*

Some people like to shave their asses because they like the way it looks, others say that a shaved ass is a more sensitive ass. Besides its practical use, many people find that shaving their own or their partners' genitals can be very erotic. Guidelines for shaving the anal area are very similar to those for shaving other pubic areas, like pussies, cocks, and balls. Find a clean, well-lit place to do it. Shaving your own ass can be difficult, so either enlist your partner to help or use a mirror so you can see what you're doing. Apply a nonirritating shaving cream or

High heels put your ass on a pedestal—where it belongs.

—Valerie Steele—

gel (as with my soap recommendations, avoid scented creams or gels which can be irritating to genitals). Use a clean, new disposable razor; choose a double- or triple-blade razor for the closest shave. Begin slowly, shaving in the direction of the hair growth. Use your other hand to pull the skin taut and prevent nicks or scrapes. Rinse the area well. As the hair grows back, it will itch. Most people who shave regularly say that the itching greatly decreases the more you do it. Try witch hazel for the itching. If you use lotion or vitamin A & D ointment to soothe the itch, make sure to wipe it off and then wash your ass before penetration, since these products usually contain oils, which will break down latex condoms and toys. Never use hair removal creams (brands like Nair) in the genital area.

Ask the Anal Advisor: *Anal Hair Removal*

Q: *Have you ever known of anyone using electrolysis or laser hair removal on their butt? Would it be safe and effective?*

A: In electrolysis, an electrical current is used to destroy the hair follicle. There is a certain amount of pain with any electrolysis (some people describe it as a slight needle prick or a quick burning sensation), and because your anal area is sensitive to begin with, there's probably more pain from the procedure there than, say, on your legs. Electrolysis treats one hair follicle at a time and requires multiple treatment sessions on each follicle to achieve a permanent result. Laser hair removal uses an infrared laser light directed at the hair. The light energy is absorbed by the pigment melanin, which then is transformed into heat energy to disable the hair follicle. A laser can treat hundreds of hairs at a time, so it can take less time than electrolysis. Laser treatment is less painful, but does not work on everyone, especially people with darker skin. The best results are achieved on people with fair skin around the ass and dark hair. It does not work on people with light-colored pubic hair or people whose hair and skin are close in color. Both laser treatment and electrolysis are expensive; however, they are both permanent after several (about four or five) treatments. It's an investment in time and money and there are risks associated with both procedures. If these procedures interest you, do some research, and contact a licensed dermatologist or cosmetologist for a consultation.

Messy and more painful than shaving, waxing your ass generally lasts longer. While I know some folks who do their own waxing at home, I say leave it to the people who do it for a living. Find a licensed professional at a reputable salon that comes recommended by someone you know. Be prepared for it to hurt, like ripping a Band-Aid off your butthole. Your ass may be tender and a little swollen right after the procedure. Don't get waxed right before an anal sex date; give your ass a day or two to recover.

NOTE

1. Chloe, in Tristan Taormino's video, *Tristan Taormino's Ultimate Guide to Anal Sex for Women* (Evil Angel, 1999).

QUOTE

Valerie Steele, *Shoes: A Lexicon of Style* (London: Scriptum Editions, 1998).

5

Enemas

An enema is the process of introducing water (or another liquid solution) into the rectum to flush out the colon, rectum, and anal canal. As the water makes its way into your ass, it loosens fecal matter and stimulates the bowels. Although you don't need to have an enema in order to have relatively safe and clean anal sex, some people prefer it. If you're going to have lots of anal sex in one session or are planning to try large toys or fisting, then I definitely recommend an enema. For people who might be squeamish about any potential mess, an enema will not only clean their ass, but also give them reassurance and confidence.

As a solo activity, an enema can be accomplished relatively quickly, or you can take some time as part of an overall pre-sex ritual, where you bathe, shave, and prepare your body and mind for a hot date. This can serve not only to cleanse the body, but also to help ground you, help you meditate and think about what's coming. It can also be something you share with your partner in preparation for a sexual experience. Some people enjoy giving or receiving enemas; they may get sexual pleasure from the sensations an enema produces, the intimacy the process creates, or the taboo nature of doing anything involving bodily functions. (See chapter 13 for a discussion of erotic enema play.)

Whether by yourself or with someone, you can give (or take) an enema anywhere you feel comfortable. If you do it in the bathroom, when you feel the urge to go, you don't have to go very far. You may feel more comfortable lying on a bed. Wherever you do it, make sure you are close to the bathroom. This chapter will cover three different types of enemas: plastic bottle and bulb syringe, enema bag, and shower attachment.

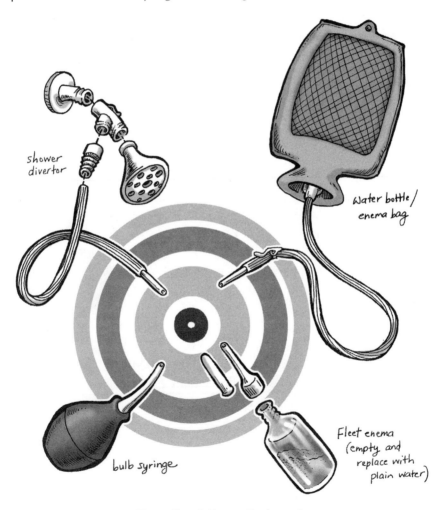

shower divertor

Water bottle / enema bag

bulb syringe

Fleet enema (empty and replace with plain water)

Illustration 4: Enema Equipment

Plastic Bottle and Bulb Syringe Enemas

The two simplest kinds of enemas are a disposable plastic bottle enema available at drug stores and a reusable rubber bulb syringe you can purchase on various websites. Inexpensive and easy to find, they require no set up or additional equipment, so you can use them nearly anywhere, and they're easy to travel with. Because they hold a relatively small amount of water, these kinds of enemas generally clean out the anal canal and lower rectum; they won't get into the upper rectum or colon to give you the deepest clean, but they are quick and simple to use.

The most commonly known brand of plastic bottle enema is the Fleet enema, which you can find at most drugstores; less expensive generic versions are also available. To use it, unscrew the plastic top and pour out the contents. All store-bought enemas contain a chemical laxative, which you don't need. Rinse the bottle several times and refill it with plain warm water. Cool or cold water can produce discomfort and cramping, so make sure the water is warm enough. The water should feel warm to the touch, but never hot or scalding (recommendations are for a temperature between 100–105°F). Replace the top on the plastic bottle, then remove the cover of the nozzle tip. Most nozzle tips come prelubricated, but feel free to add some of your favorite lube to make insertion easier.

Pick a comfortable position that allows you easy access to your ass. You can squat over the toilet, lean over the edge of the bathtub, kneel with your ass up and shoulders down, or lay on your side with one leg up. Gently slide the nozzle tip of the bottle into your ass. Squeeze the bottle to release the water into your butt. Take a deep breath, and see if you can hold the water. The amount of time you can hold the water varies from person to person; it may be anywhere from a few seconds to a few minutes. Your body will tell you when it's time to sit on the toilet and have a bowel movement. Refill the bottle, and repeat the steps until all that comes out of your ass is clear water. Since the standard plastic bottle enema holds only 4.5 ounces, you may also choose to fill the bottle, fill your ass, then refill the bottle and your ass a few times until you feel full, then evacuate. After you're done, you should discard the bottle since it's made for single use only.

Bulb syringes are made of a thicker, more durable rubber and hold twice as much water as a plastic bottle (the standard size is 10 ounces);

some also come with interchangeable nozzles. The bulb syringe works the same way as the plastic bottle except that it does not come prefilled and it's reusable. Follow the instructions above. When you are finished, clean the syringe and nozzle with hot water and antibacterial soap and let it dry completely.

Few generals or presid
ever exercise such personal
power as a nurse and her
enema bag do in controlling
the bowels of a patient.
—DR. JERRY GLENN KNOX —

Enema Bags and Accessories

If you'd like to have an enema that cleans the entire rectum as well as the colon, choose an enema bag. Compared to plastic bottle enemas and bulb syringes, an enema bag takes more equipment, more time, and a little more skill. The equipment is still portable, although it will take up more room in your luggage if you travel. The advantage of an enema bag is that you can fill your rectum with more water than with a bottle or syringe.

The easiest way to purchase an enema bag setup is to get a kit that includes all the necessary items: bag, tubing, clamp, nozzle, and hook. You can also purchase these items separately at medical and fetish websites (see Resource Guide). Here's a guide to the necessary items:

BAGS: The most recognizable and available enema bag is the red rubber 2-quart bag, sold in most drug stores with all the necessary accessories. You can find this and other rubber bags as well as silicone bags at specialty stores and websites. Silicone is a lot more expensive than rubber, but it's much more resilient since it is not affected by typical wear and tear like rubber is. Silicone bags will last a long time, whereas rubber bags should be replaced every few years. Enema bags come in a variety of colors and sizes, including 2 quart, 4 quart, and 5 quart.

TUBING: Tubing that connects the enema bag to the nozzle can be made of latex rubber or silicone. It comes in a variety of colors and some different widths, although 5/16" is the most common.

CLAMPS: Made of plastic or metal, the clamp is what controls the flow of water from the bag through the tube and into your ass. An *on/off* clamp offers only one speed, so you cannot control the flow of the water. A ratchet-type clamp gives you much better control of the flow, but going from *on* to *off* isn't immediate. Some folks like to use two clamps: one near the bag that has a flow control, and one closer to the nozzle that's *on/off*. That way, you can experiment with water speed, and once you decide on

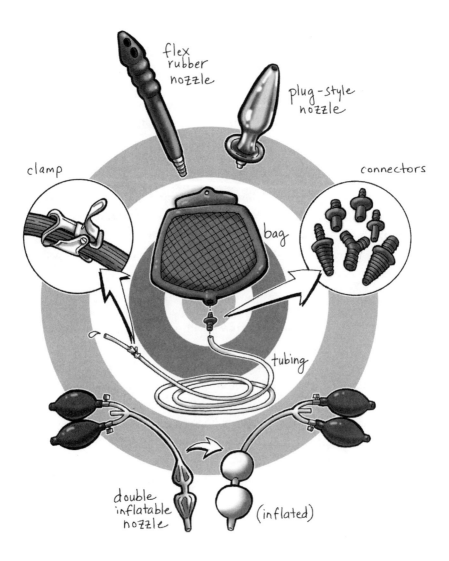

Illustration 5: Enema Bag Equipment and Nozzles

speed, set the ratchet, then set the *on/off* clamp to *off*. When you switch it to *on*, you've got your desired speed.

CONNECTORS: The advantage to buying an enema kit is that everything fits together. If you buy your items separately, not everything may be the same size, since widths of enema bag openings, tubing, and nozzles can vary from 1/4" to 5/16" to 3/4". If the items you want to use are not the same size, then you need connectors. For example, in order to use a bag with a 1/4" opening and tubing that's 5/16" together, you need a 1/4"-to-5/16" connector. Connectors are sold separately at enema equipment specialty stores and websites.

HOOKS: Enema kits come with a plastic hook or you can purchase one separately. This is a small but important piece since you'll need to hang the enema bag.

TOWELS: It's a good idea to put a bath mat down on the floor, and have a towel or two nearby. If you're administering an enema to yourself or someone else in a place other than a bathroom, you may want to lay down towels or absorbent bed pads.

FLOW INDICATORS: Although not necessary for an effective enema, a flow indicator is a cool accessory for enema fans. Flow indicators attach to the enema tubing and measure the speed of the water flow.

Enema Nozzles

When you purchase an enema bag kit, it comes with a basic nozzle for the end of the tubing; it's made of a firmer material than the tubing and has one or more holes in it through which the water flows. If you purchase your enema items separately, you'll definitely need to get a nozzle. Since the nozzle is the part that goes inside your ass, you want the size, shape, and material to be comfortable for you. Here are some examples of different kinds (also see Illustration 5):

FLEXIBLE RUBBER NOZZLES: These slim, soft rubber nozzles are easy to insert and great for enema beginners. Because they're skinny, though, some people complain that water can leak out more easily.

HARD RUBBER OR PLASTIC NOZZLES: These small but hard nozzles are often sold in a set of several different sizes and shapes. Their size is good for novices, although their firmness may be less comfortable than a more flexible material.

BUTT PLUG STYLE NOZZLES: Made of a variety of materials including rubber, hard plastic, aluminum, and stainless steel, these nozzles look like butt plugs and anal bead toys because basically they are—except they attach to tubing and have holes in the tips for water to flow through. If you want to add a pleasurable element to your enema, then nozzles that "double" as toys are for you.

INFLATABLE BALLOON NOZZLES: The top-of-the-line accessories that enema aficionados rave about are the single and double inflatable balloon nozzles. Picture a rubber arrow-shaped nozzle with an inflator bulb attached. The idea behind the design is that once you insert and inflate the nozzle, it forms a kind of seal which helps you keep it in. They can be very expensive (from one-hundred to two-hundred dollars), but they are worth it. There are also less expensive disposable models on the market.

For the single inflatable, lube up the deflated nozzle and carefully insert it into the ass. Since it's so squishy, getting it in can be a challenge. Try twisting it back and forth or slipping a finger under the bottom of the nozzle to help guide it. Once it's in, inflate the balloon with several squeezes of the inflator bulb (about one to four squeezes for 250cc balloons and one to eight for the larger variety). Once the balloon is inflated, tug on it very gently to make sure that it is sitting just inside the inner sphincters.

One complaint about the single balloon nozzle is that it can shift position and water can leak past it. The double inflatable has two nozzles designed to solve this problem: one sits just inside the sphincter and the other sits outside the anal opening to hold everything in place. Insert the first nozzle, following the single nozzle instructions above. Once that nozzle is in and inflated, inflate the second nozzle just outside the anus. Once the nozzles are in place and feel snug, you can begin the flow of water.

Inflatable nozzles come in rubber and silicone; never use oil-based lubes on rubber, or silicone lubes on silicone. For cleaning instructions, see the cleaning section later in this chapter.

Ask the Anal Advisor: *Sit-on Enema Bag*

Q: *I saw a picture of an enema bag on the Internet that looked like a hot water bottle that you sit on. Have you ever heard of such a thing?*

A: Modeled after enema bag designs from the 1920s, the "sit-on" enema bag looks like a whoopee cushion with a butt plug nozzle in the center. You literally sit on the nozzle and your body weight forces the water into your ass. No tube, no clamp. It sounds like it wouldn't work, especially since you're working against gravity in this situation, but the folks I know who've used it simply love it. This kind of enema bag is hard to find, so I recommend BethTyler.com.

Using an Enema Bag

One you've got all your equipment and the appropriate pieces are connected to one another, you're almost ready to start your enema. Fill the bag with plain warm water. Test the temperature on your wrist first to make sure it's not too hot. If you're going to fuss with things for several minutes after you fill the bag, then you can make the water slightly hotter and it will cool off. It's best to fill the bag entirely, even if you don't think you'll take the whole thing, to prevent air bubbles.

Hang the enema bag approximately 18–24" from where your butt will be when you get into your desired position. This could be on the shower curtain rod, on a hook, or if you're very fancy, on an IV stand. The idea here is that gravity powers the enema, so it needs to be far enough above you to work but not so high up that the water flows too quickly. When the bag is full—before you insert anything—unlock the clamp and let the water begin to flow into the tub, sink, or a bucket. You can make sure everything is properly connected and working, and you can adjust the flow if your clamp is ratchet-style. This also allows you to release any air bubbles. Close the clamp.

If you're giving yourself an enema, make sure the clamp is close enough to the nozzle to be within easy reach for you. You can proceed two ways: insert the well-lubricated nozzle into your ass, then get into the position you want to be in, or get into position, then insert the nozzle.

This, along with your chosen position, is something you should experiment with beforehand to see what's comfortable. If you're using a nozzle bigger than the size of a finger, you need to warm up the ass with fingers or smaller toys before you put it in. Some people like to lie on their back with their knees up and hips tilted forward for easy access; others prefer to lay on their stomachs or in a fetal position. You could get into doggie-style position or on your knees with ass up and head down, especially if someone is helping you with your enema. The traditional position used in hospitals is lying on your left side with your right leg pulled up to your chest. Standing up, sitting up, or squatting are the trickiest positions because the colon is not in the best position for gravity to work its magic, but if this position works for you, then go for it. When you're ready, unlock the clamp to begin the flow of water. If the clamp is adjustable, begin with the lowest flow speed at first. You can always increase it later, but the lowest is absolutely recommended for beginners.

Take some deep breaths as the water fills your ass. It's going to feel strange at first. Since your rectum is used to expelling matter, having water flow into it, however slowly, can feel a little weird at first. Don't worry—this sensation of fullness in your rectum just takes some getting used to. You may feel uncomfortable at first, but it should not feel painful at all. If you experience any cramping, close the clamp and take some deep breaths. Try changing positions or bringing the bag closer to you. Proceed when you feel ready.

Experts agree that the average person can take about 2 quarts of water. But an average is just that, so take as much or as little as you can. Experienced enemates shouldn't take more than 4 quarts at one time, although even larger-sized bags are sold and people do use them safely. You'll know when you've had enough because you'll have the sensation of fullness and pressure or you'll have the urge to go the bathroom. At this point, some people are able to take a deep breath and relax and take in some more. Others need to stop. Do what works for you. When you're ready to stop, close the clamp. When you're full, hold the water for as long as feels comfortable. This could be a few seconds or a few minutes, depending on your experience and comfort level. You'll have a distinct urge to have a bowel movement; listen to your body. Carefully slide the nozzle out of your ass, sit on the toilet, and let nature takes its course. I prefer to leave the nozzle in until the last moment, so I detach the nozzle from the tubing (whatever water remains in the tube from the clamp to the nozzle will come out, so be prepared for that), sit on the toilet, then slide the nozzle out once I'm there. You can do it either way.

Give yourself plenty of time to evacuate. When you go, it may feel like having diarrhea. That's normal since you've just introduced a lot of water into the rectum and loosened everything up. When you're done, you may decide to go a second round. In that case, repeat the steps until only clear water comes out of your ass. When it's over, clean your enema equipment and drink a glass of water or a sports drink to stay hydrated.

Shower Attachment Enemas

A guy I know from Texas installed an enema attachment in his shower. Shortly thereafter, his mother came to his house. Notoriously nosey, she snooped around, as she usually did, looking into every nook and cranny and inspecting his cleaning skills. During her visit to his bathroom, although the shower curtain was closed, she pulled it back to check out the bathtub. When she came out of the bathroom, she asked, "What's that fancy thing in the shower for?" Caught off guard and more than a little embarrassed, he answered quickly, "Oh, that's for giving the dog a bath."

"What a great idea!" she responded. "You'll have to install one in my house!" Not wanting to get caught in a lie, the next weekend he installed a Shower Shot enema attachment for his mother. Either she's figured out what it's really for, or that's one clean dog she's got.

You can buy an attachment for your shower—called the nozzle attachment, shower diverter, Shower Shot, or the Shur Shot—through some hardware stores or at specialty retail websites. The attachment diverts the water from the shower head to a hose with a nozzle at the end of it. Some systems allow water to flow through both the shower head and the nozzle, so you can have an enema and get the rest of you body clean simultaneously. Some are made entirely of chrome-plated brass and metal, others are made of chrome with vinyl hoses and plastic nozzles. Some shower attachment sets come with a nozzle, others do not; a wide variety of nozzles—including aluminum butt plug style nozzles, stainless steel interchangeable nozzles, and jelly dong nozzles—are sold separately. Some diverters are a simple *on/off* style, while others are a combination of *on/off* and a flow control.

The upside to this type of enema is the convenience and a constant water supply—no bag to refill, no pieces to assemble; your enema setup is right there in the shower. You also have much more control over the water flow, which is controlled by the faucets in your tub. You can often take as much or more water as you can with an enema bag, for a deeper cleaning. The downside is you can't take it with you anywhere you go! There are a few things that are important to consider before you decide to invest in one of these attachment kits (which usually cost from forty to seventy dollars). You should only use a shower attachment if you have good control over your water temperature and pressure. If you live in an apartment building where either regularly fluctuates, or in a house with older plumbing or a small hot water heater, this is not the enema setup for you. If, during a shower, you often find the water going from the perfect temperature to freezing or scalding in an instant, then yours is not the ideal shower for an enema attachment.

> He's told her that it's a natural human need, this ritual. He's emphasized...[the] sense of regression, of being small, cared for, looked after...all thoughts she'll feel as he bares her behind, spreads her cheeks, puts the nozzle in, opens the clamp. And rubs between her legs as she squirms and shifts over his lap, feeling the pressure in her bowels grow.
> —M. R. STRICT—

If you're a good candidate, then purchase an attachment kit and follow the instructions to install it. After installation, it's best to test things out before you christen it. Set the water temperature and pressure to a comfortable level. Flip the lever that switches the flow and see how it works. Once you're satisfied with the setup, you can begin. Find a comfortable position; since you're in the shower you may want to stand or kneel and lean over the edge of the tub. Lubricate the nozzle, and warm up your ass first. Just as with an enema bag enema, you're going to fill up, hold it, and evacuate. Some people get out of the shower and sit on the toilet, while others prefer to stay right in the shower. Doing it right in the shower means you don't have to keep jumping in and out; however, you should only release the water (and everything that comes with it) from your ass into the shower if you know that you've got an exceptional drainage system. Believe me, you don't want to call a plumber in the middle of your enema. Repeat the enema until you're all clean.

Enema Do's and Don'ts

Giving enemas is a skill that takes practice and patience. You should feel only a little discomfort during an enema; if you experience pain or cramping, go sit on the toilet right away. Allow yourself plenty of time and several bowel movements before you're cleaned out. If you are a frequent enema-taker or are concerned about losing electrolytes, you can add 1 teaspoon of sea salt per 1 quart of water. The salt brings the enema water more closely in balance with bodily fluids and helps prevent too much water from being absorbed by the colon. When less water is absorbed, you can get a better cleansing, and more water will come out of your ass. You may also feel the need to pee less often.

You should finish an enema at least two to three hours before you plan to have anal sex. This time gives your body a chance to recover and allows the thin layer of mucous that lines and protects the rectum to regenerate. Plus, it prevents another potential situation. Sometimes, I believe I'm all done with my enema. I get dressed to run some errands. Inevitably, I wait on some impossibly long line at the post office or somewhere, and just as I get to the counter, I have an urge. Oh. My. God. My enema is so not over. This is what I call the "second wave" (the discovery that there was more in there), and the second wave can happen without warning. If the second wave happens in the middle of an anal sex date, then things are going to be messier than if you never had an enema in the first place. So give yourself plenty of time between enema and anal sex.

People with high blood pressure, heart problems, serious health conditions, or a compromised immune system should talk to a doctor before having an enema. Even if you're in good health, it's not a good idea to have enemas too frequently. They tend to stress out your rectum, and too much of this evacuation can throw your rectum, bowels, and gastrointestinal tract off balance. There is no agreed-upon frequency, but I will say this: once a day every day is too much, once a month is fine. Once a week or every two weeks is okay as long as it's not every single week—give yourself some longer breaks. Do not overdo it on enemas. I don't want to see any of you at an Enema Addicts Anonymous meeting! If, after an enema, you don't have a bowel movement or expel any liquid, you could be dehydrated or have a serious condition. See a doctor immediately.

Enema Tips

- If you don't trust your tap water (for example, if you wouldn't drink it), use bottled distilled water, and warm it up before you fill the syringe or enema bag.

- Never use a vaginal douche in your rectum.

- Do not share enema equipment.

- Always clean your enema equipment carefully right after you use it.

- Read and follow all instructions that accompany enema kits or equipment.

Cleaning Enema Equipment

One way to clean rubber or silicone enema bags, tubing, and nozzles is to wash them thoroughly with warm water and antibacterial soap or soak them in a soap and water solution, then rinse them several times with plain water. Make sure to dry all items completely, especially the bag, so no mold or mildew forms on surfaces.

There are differences of opinion when it comes to using bleach to clean enema equipment. Some people recommend soaking both rubber and silicone equipment in a diluted bleach solution (10 parts water, 1 part bleach) for about 20 minutes. Rinse all items, especially the bag, several times to make sure no bleach remains and dry them properly. Others caution that a thorough rinse is not enough, and some bleach will likely remain on the equipment. The next time you have an enema, this theory goes, that bleach will end up in your ass.

Because of gravity, there's no chance that fecal matter can travel from your ass into the enema bag, so as long as the bag is rinsed out (even in only hot water) and properly dried, it will be fine. Bacteria and fecal matter from the ass can get on nozzles and even migrate from nozzles to tubing, so if you're going to be anal retentive about cleaning, those are the items you should concentrate on. Whether you use a mild soap (and cotton swabs or pipe cleaners to make sure to get in nooks and crannies) or a bleach solution, the most important step is rinse, rinse, rinse.

Remember that rubber items are porous and can never be completely disinfected. Silicone isn't porous, and can be disinfected with hot water and antibacterial soap, although I still recommend that you never share enema equipment with another person. Nozzles made of other materials should be cleaned according to their specific instructions (Also see the guidelines for toy cleaning in chapter 8).

Inflatable nozzles require extra care when cleaning and storing. Heat, direct sunlight, dampness, and harsh chemicals will all degrade them and shorten their shelf life. Wash the nozzle and its connecting tube in warm water and a mild soap. Be especially careful not to get any water in the air tubes or the inflators since this will ruin them. Use a towel to dry off, making sure it's completely dry, then dust it lightly with cornstarch and store it in a cool, dry, dark place.

Enema Ingredients

Some of you may have heard about oil enemas or various ingredients you can add to plain water enemas like soap, salt, or various herbal remedies. Any and all of these can irritate the lining of the rectum, which is very delicate. Any substance that you introduce into the rectum gets absorbed very quickly and goes directly into the bloodstream. It's not the same as ingesting the exact substance because when we eat or drink something, it has the benefit of going through our stomachs and livers where it's broken down before it enters the bloodstream.

I'm a purist when it comes to enemas. I believe that plain warm water does a fine job, and that the risks are too great for a negative reaction from adding other ingredients (except sea salt to balance electrolytes as previously discussed). I include the most popular kinds of enemas in this chapter for informational purposes, but I do not endorse them. I suggest you consult a health care professional before you do any kind of enema other than a plain water one.

Soap is probably the most common thing people add to an enema. While I see the logical connection between soap and cleaning, the point of an enema is to flush out fecal matter, not wash it like dirty feet. You should never use liquid antibacterial soap, body wash, or dishwashing detergent as they are too harsh; castile soap is the gentlest of all liquid soaps. Enema equipment retailers often carry castile soap and some enema practitioners extol the virtues of soap enemas. You should use only a few drops of soap in the water, and do several plain enemas after to rinse thoroughly. No matter how mild the soap, it can still irritate the delicate tissue of the rectum, which is why I caution against it.

Oil has been used over the years for its laxative properties and can be helpful in relieving constipation or what Certified Colon Hydrotherapist Kristina Amelong calls "a sluggish colon."[2] Vegetable oil, olive oil, castor oil, or mineral oil can stimulate the defecation process, but again, if you're in good health and simply want to flush out your ass, you don't need oil to do it. Besides an oil enema is a chore to clean up after.

Herbal remedies like chamomile, peppermint, fennel, aloe vera, lavender, and dozens of others are used in enemas for their various healing properties, to stimulate immune function, or to treat specific medical conditions. Just because these ingredients are natural doesn't automatically mean they are safe. Consult a medical professional before using any of them orally or rectally.

Coffee enemas are said to have a detoxifying effect on the liver, gall bladder, and other organs, and some people swear by coffee enemas for good health. Be aware that coffee can also be an irritant, and because it

Ask the Anal Advisor: *Wild Weekend*

Q: *I am visiting my lover for a four-day weekend, and, since we don't see each other very often, we plan to have lots of sex, including plenty of anal penetration. I want to be clean for the entire time, so can I have an enema every day?*

A: Having an enema every day of your four-day romp will probably do more harm than good. Enemas stress out the body, and too many enemas in such a short period of time can disrupt the production of mucous to protect the rectum and definitely throw things off balance. Here's my recommendation: have a nice-sized enema (with an enema bag or shower attachment) the night before you arrive. That should keep you cleaned out for several days, provided you eat a healthy diet and have regular bowel movements. By day three, if you want to clean again, do a rinse with a plastic bottle or bulb syringe—it will reassure you that you're still clean, without overdoing it.

contains caffeine, a stimulant. Like other ingredients, I don't recommend it unless you're under the supervision of a health care provider.

Alcohol enemas of any kind—wine, beer, or hard liquor—not only irritate rectal tissue like other substances, but are extremely dangerous. Because of the amazing absorptive quality of the rectum, putting something in your ass is like shooting it directly into your veins. It bypasses the stomach and liver, and goes straight to the bloodstream. Alcohol dehydrogenase (ADH), the enzyme that breaks down alcohol after you drink it, is present in the stomach and liver, but very little in the colon. Normally, alcohol is partially metabolized in the liver before it hits your bloodstream and you start feeling its effects. With an alcohol enema, not only are the effects felt almost immediately, but the amount of alcohol it takes to get you intoxicated is much less. In addition to making you sick, alcohol enemas, even when diluted with water, can lead to alcohol poisoning.

NOTE

1. Kristina Amelong on www.optimalhealthnetwork.com.

QUOTES

Dr. Jerry Glenn Knox, *Love Thine Enemas & Heal Thyself* (Vancouver, WA: Lifeknox Publishing, 2002), 15.

M. R. Strict, *Intimate Invasions: The Erotic Ins and Outs of Enema Play* (Oakland, CA: Greenery Press, 2004), 2.

Safer Sex

Every sexual encounter we have with another person has its own physical and emotional risks, responsibilities, and rewards. While we may not be able to anticipate or guard against feelings or issues that arise from an erotic experience, we can protect our bodies from infection and disease. It's important to know what STDs or sexually transmitted diseases (also known as STIs or sexually transmitted infections) are, how they are transmitted, and how to protect ourselves from them. I cover the most common STDs—human papillomavirus, genital herpes, chlamydia, gonorrhea, syphilis, hepatitis, and HIV/AIDS—in chapter 17. It's equally important for you and your partner to get tested regularly for STDs regardless of your sexual orientation. Unless you and your partner are monogamous and have recently tested negative for all STDs, you may be at risk to give or get an STD. Practicing safer sex can decrease the chances of STD transmission.

It's a good idea to practice safer sex if: you or your partner have an STD; you don't know your own or your partner's STD status; or you are not in a monogamous relationship with an STD-free partner. Here are some of the tools you can use to protect yourself and your partner.

ASK THE ANAL ADVISOR: *Rash from Her Ass*

Q: *I recently started dating, well, fucking, somebody I've known for close to a year. She has been without a sexual partner for a long time, but she's a serious hypochondriac about STDs; she was tested for everything twice in April, and once last month. She gets depo shots, so we fuck without condoms. So, how come I get a strange rash on my glans and foreskin, usually lasting for a day or two, when I fuck her in the ass? It doesn't hurt and it basically just makes the regular bumps and pores looks bigger and red. There's no funky smell or discharge either. I've studied the symptoms of about every friggin' STD more than this girl has, plus I've been tested more than she has. It doesn't look like any STD I've heard of.*

A: I know you think your lover is a hypochondriac, but I applaud both of you for getting tested often because most people do not. And it also sounds like you know a lot about STDs, which makes you more educated than the average guy on that subject. You may be having an allergic reaction to the lube you are using. Most lubes, whether water-based or silicone-based have similar ingredients, but they are not all the same. Personally, I got a red, itchy pussy from one particular brand of lube that I was trying out for the first time. I never used it again, and I haven't had the symptoms again. So, try using a different brand of lube and see if that changes anything. You could also go to your doctor when you're having symptoms to get a full examination and see what he or she has to say. It sounds like you know a lot about STDs, but it's always better to be safe than sorry.

Gloves

Putting a glove on your hand for rubbing and finger-fucking protects both you and your partner, especially if you have any cuts, scratches, or even torn cuticles, which can provide STDs direct access to your bloodstream. Gloves made of latex are the most popular and widely available, and latex is a good safer sex barrier. If, however, you are allergic or sensitive to latex, there are gloves made of other materials, including nitrile, vinyl, and neoprene. Powdered gloves make getting them on and off easier, but the powder can often irritate people's skin; if your skin feels itchy or turns red and you know you're not allergic to the glove material, find one that's not powdered.

Gloves come in several different sizes, from extra small to extra large, and it's important to find the right size for your hand. A glove that's too small will cut off your circulation and have a greater risk of tearing. One that is too big gives the wearer less sensitivity, and can feel baggy and uncomfortable to the receptive partner. Besides being great for safer sex, gloves can also reassure you—if your nails are long or ragged, if you or your partner are squeamish about the cleanliness of anal penetration, or if you want to smooth out your fingers before they go inside your lover. When you wear a glove, always use plenty of lube to reduce friction and make penetration smoother.

Oral Sex Barriers

To protect you and your partner during oral-anal contact, you can use one of several safer sex barriers. The most popular is a latex dental dam. Originally designed for use by dentists (as the name indicates), dental dams are squares of latex that safer sex practitioners have co-opted for use as oral sex barriers. Because they were not developed with sex in mind, dental dams can be too small and too thick to make them ideal. Several companies—like Glyde, Slicks, Lixx, and Good Vibrations—have improved upon the dental dam, designing larger, thinner dams specifically for oral sex that do the job much better than their traditional counterparts. Hot Dam makes polyurethane dams for those allergic to latex. Some dams come scented or flavored, and most are available at better sex toy stores.

To make your own dam out of a latex or nonlatex glove, you can cut a nonlubricated condom up one side; these tend to be thinner like the Glydes, allowing both partners more feeling and greater sensitivity. You can also transform a latex glove into a dam (see illustration 6): Cut the wrist and the fingers off, leaving the thumb intact, then cut up the side where the pinkie was. Open it up, stick your tongue in the thumb slot, and voilà—it's like a condom for your tongue! This is my favorite kind of dam because it affords both giver and receiver the highest sensitivity. For obvious reasons, it's best to use a glove that isn't powdered or to rinse the powder off before you put your mouth near it. Try putting a dab of lube on the inside and outside of the thumb for even more sensitivity.

Store-bought plastic wrap (brands like Saran Wrap) is not just for left-overs—it also makes a good barrier for rimming. Plastic wrap is less expensive and easier to find than latex dams, which makes it more convenient. Another advantage: it can cover a lot more surface area and no one has to hold the dam in place. Try wrapping your sweetie's privates in plastic—think of it as a homemade thong for safe, hands-free ass licking. You can simply cut it off when you're all done.

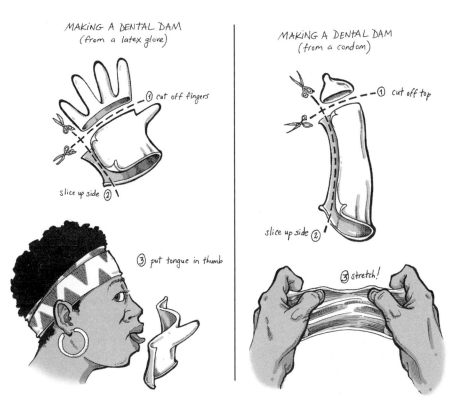

Illustration 6: Making a Dental Dam

Anal Activities and STD Risks

RUBBING: *manual external stimulation with fingers, without penetration, without a glove.* At risk for genital warts, genital herpes; if skin of fingers or skin of the anus is broken, at risk for chlamydia, gonorrhea, syphilis, hepatitis B.

FINGERING: *anal penetration with a finger or fingers without a glove.* At risk for genital warts, genital herpes; if skin of fingers or skin of the anus or anal canal is broken, at risk for chlamydia, gonorrhea, syphilis, hepatitis B, hepatitis C, HIV.

LICKING: *analingus or rimming without a barrier.* At risk for genital warts, genital herpes, chlamydia, gonorrhea, syphilis, hepatitis A; if open sores on anus or in anal canal, at risk for hepatitis B, hepatitis C, HIV.

ANAL INTERCOURSE: *anal penetration with a penis, without a condom, with or without ejaculation.* At risk for genital warts, genital herpes, chlamydia, gonorrhea, syphilis, hepatitis B, hepatitis C, HIV.

ANAL INTERCOURSE WITH CONDOM: *anal penetration with a penis, with a condom, with or without ejaculation.* At risk for genital warts, genital herpes, syphilis.

SHARING SEX TOYS: *transferring a sex toy from an infected person's orifice to another person's orifice without putting a condom on it or disinfecting it first.* At risk for chlamydia, gonorrhea, hepatitis B, hepatitis C, HIV.

Condoms

If someone is going to stick his dick in your ass, and you are practicing safer sex, he should use a condom. Because of the delicacy of anal and rectal tissue (which may lead to minute tears), semen infected with HIV and other STDs can be transmitted and absorbed easier and more quickly into the bloodstream. Thus, unprotected anal intercourse can be more risky for both partners than unprotected vaginal intercourse. There are dozens of brands and varieties of condoms on the market, and finding the right one for you could mean trying a bunch out until you find one you love. The majority of condoms are made of latex, but people with latex allergies or sensitivities should try alternative materials like polyurethane from brands like Durex Avanti and Trojan Supra (only available with spermicide). Trojan Naturalambs, unique condoms made from lamb intestines, do not prevent STDs.

These days, there are lots of condoms on the market with fancy bells and whistles: ribbed; studded; ridged, for her pleasure, for his pleasure, or both. Condoms with stimulating textures on the inside ("for his pleasure") are totally safe for anal penetration. Condoms with stimulating textures on the outside ("for her pleasure") may cause irritation or minute abrasions to the rectal tissue. Some people say that the texture is so subtle, they don't notice a difference, while others claim that textured condoms are uncomfortable. The newest design on the market is one with a baggier head to increase sensitivity for the head of the penis; these condoms (popular brands include InSpiral and Trojan Twisted) are safe for anal intercourse, but some may find they make insertion more difficult.

Most condoms come prelubricated, but you can also buy nonlubed condoms; either way, you can add your own favorite lube. You should never use a condom lubricated with nonoxynol-9. Nonoxynol-9, which is found in some lubricants and some lubricated condoms, is a chemical proven to kill the HIV virus and STDs in laboratory tests. Although it was once widely recommended that nonoxynol-9 be used for safer sex, we now know that many people are allergic to nonoxynol-9 and it really irritates their vaginas and rectums. Because it is so harsh for the delicate tissue of the ass, research has shown that it's more likely to irritate or traumatize the rectal tissue, which can actually make transmission of HIV faster and easier, providing the virus with an accessible route to the bloodstream. Read condom labels to make sure the lube does not contain nonoxynol-9.

When used correctly, condoms are highly effective in preventing STD transmission; *correctly* is the key word here (see illustration 7). There are more untrustworthy people than there are untrustworthy condoms. Three important elements will help ensure a condom's effectiveness: fit, putting it on properly, and taking it off properly. Fit is incredibly important not only for the sensitivity of both partners, but also for safety. A condom that fits well is less likely to slip off or to break. Each brand of condoms fits each penis slightly differently. Brands like Exotica Snugger Fit or LifeStyles Snugger Fit offer smaller sizes, and popular larger size brands include Durex XXL, Kimono Maxx, LifeStyles XL, and Trojan Magnum and Magnum XL.

Putting on a condom the right way is very important. First, make sure it's not inside out. If you use a condom with a receptacle tip, gently press the air out of the closed end before putting it on. Air bubbles can rupture condoms. If you use a condom with a plain end, leave about an inch of air-free space at the tip of the condom; semen needs somewhere to go and ejaculation without that space can cause a condom to break. Putting a small amount of lube on the inside tip of the condom will reduce air bubbles and increase sensitivity.

If your partner has ejaculated during penetration, whether he feels his erection has gone down a little, all the way, or not at all, he should hold on to the base of the condom as he withdraws. By not holding on, he runs the risk of coming out without the condom; then he or you have to fish around inside your ass for it, which is both awkward and unsafe, since semen could spill out of the condom. If he feels himself losing his erection during penetration or he withdraws before ejaculation, he should also hold on to the base.

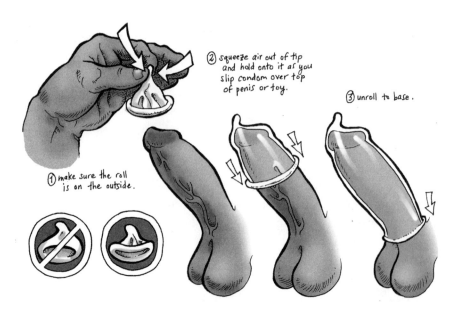

② squeeze air out of tip and hold onto it as you slip condom over top of penis or toy.

③ unroll to base.

① make sure the roll is on the outside.

Illustration 7: Putting on a Condom

The Female Condom

Marketed primarily for vaginal intercourse, the Reality Female Condom˙ is a tube of polyurethane closed at one end and open at the other, like a larger version of the male condom. Although some women find them cumbersome, others say it gives them a sense of control and responsibility in the practice of safer sex. The female condom can also be used for anal intercourse, and, in fact, it offers more protection because it lines the anal cavity, covering the penis and the outer area of the anus. Some people also use the female condom for anal-oral contact, although its effectiveness for analingus has not been scientifically tested or proven. You should not use it for anal fisting. The female condom can be slipped into the ass any time before penetration. Before insertion, lubricate the outside of the condom, and make sure that the lubrication is evenly spread by rubbing the sides of the pouch together. To insert it, squeeze the sheath, and, starting with the inner ring, slip it into the anus. Make sure that the

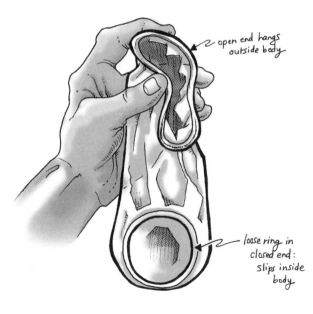

open end hangs outside body

loose ring in closed end: slips inside body

Illustration 8: Female Condom

inner ring is at the closed end of the pouch. Once it is inside, push it the rest of the way in with your finger, past the sphincter muscles. About an inch of the condom should hang outside the anus, so the outer ring doesn't slip inside during the action.

During penetration, the condom may move around, either side to side or up and down. This is normal. However, if your partner's penis or dildo is long or thrusts deeply, the condom could slip all the way into the anus. If your partner withdraws completely in between thrusts, she or he could slip back inside your anus—but outside the protection of the condom. If this happens, stop and adjust the condom. Like everything else, using the female condom takes practice and patience. To take the condom out, squeeze and twist the outer ring (to keep fluid inside the pouch) and pull it out slowly and gently. Don't flush the Reality Female Condom in the toilet—throw it away.

Making Toys Safe

Transferring a sex toy from an infected person's orifice directly to another person's orifice puts you at risk for STD transmission. When it comes to making sex toy play safe, you have a few options. If a toy is porous (made of jelly, rubber, or vinyl), you should either designate it as your own, or, if you want to share it, cover it with a condom and change condoms when you change orifices or partners. If a toy is nonporous (made of silicone, acrylic, glass, or metal), you can either cover it with a condom, or you can disinfect it before using it with another orifice or partner.

To disinfect a nonporous toy, clean it with hot water and antibacterial soap, or a diluted 10:1 bleach solution; or, if it's silicone, boil it. Porous toys cannot be disinfected. For more on sex toys, see chapter 8.

Other Safety Precautions

You should never, ever put anything in the vagina that has been in the anus without thoroughly washing and disinfecting it first. Transferring rectal bacteria into the vagina can lead to yeast infections, urinary tract infections, and other ailments that will put a halt to your pussy's health and happiness. Just don't go there. If you or your partner want to use the same finger, cock, or toy in both the vagina and the ass, either use gloves and

Ask the Anal Advisor: *Ejaculating in Her Ass*

Q: *My husband and I have been married for six years. Although he has always played with my ass while we were making love, about three weeks ago, he actually put his cock in my ass. We've been doing it ever since, and it's been great! He's rather large, but we do a lot of warm-up. Generally, we do it doggie-style because I enjoy looking in the mirror and seeing him behind me pumping away. Here's my dilemma. Dennis always pulls out when he is about to come. This is very disappointing to me, and I would like to have him continue and shoot his juice into me. Would there be any problem with allowing his sperm to get into me that way? Would a fairly good amount of semen in the rectum do anything bad?*

A: If you and your husband are monogamous, and both of you have tested negative for HIV and the other STDs, then your husband can come in your ass, and it is relatively low risk for both of you. If, however, you don't have current negative test results for all these diseases, then either of you could transmit something to the other person through unprotected anal inter-course. This is true *whether he comes inside you or not*. You said you are married, but since this is the new millennium, I will not automatically assume that you are monogamous—you or your husband may have sex with multiple partners. If that is the case and for other readers out there who may be nonmonogamous, anal penetration without a condom can put both people (and especially the receptive partner) at risk for contracting STDs. The risks increase for the receptive partner if the insertive partner ejaculates, since semen has a high concentration of HIV and many of the STDs mentioned. Since you described his load as "a fairly good amount of semen," I'll remind you that what goes in must come out, so the semen may dribble out of your ass (along with all the lube you put in there), but a quick trip to the bathroom should take care of that!

condoms, and switch them before you switch orifices or wash whatever it is post-pussy and pre-ass. If a toy is porous, like jelly, rubber, or vinyl, then you need to put a condom on it before it goes in a pussy in order for it to be completely safe after it's been in someone's ass.

Protecting Yourself

Get tested for HIV and STDs regularly.

You're at higher risk if you have unprotected anal sex with your partners.

Use condoms, dental dams, gloves, and lubricants for all anal activities.

Herpes and genital warts may appear not only on but around the genitals, and condoms and dental dams will protect only the area they cover, so partners should limit their activities accordingly during outbreaks.

Safe, slow, and gentle anal sex decreases the chances of trauma to anal/rectal tissue; keep in mind, however, that you may already have minute tears or sores in the rectal lining that you don't know about.

If you and your partner are both HIV-positive, you should still practice safer sex to avoid being exposed to a different strain of the virus or transmitting opportunistic infections.

CHAPTER

7

Lubricants

Before I slide down this particular pole, let me reveal a bias: I am a firm believer that lube makes *any* sexual activity much more pleasurable. The wetter and slipperier everything is, the better. But lubricant is not just desirable for anal penetration, it's essential. Unlike the vagina, the anal canal and rectum are not self-lubricating. During anal exploration, you might find that the ass feels wet. What you're feeling is a natural mucous secretion and maybe some sweat—but neither provides enough wetness to lubricate the ass for pleasurable penetration. And spit just won't do the trick. If you're using gloves, dams, or condoms, you absolutely need lube because unlubricated latex and latex alternatives are more likely to break without lube. Whether or not you're using safer sex barriers, you want to reduce the friction to make penetration comfortable. Lube makes penetration smoother and easier for both partners, reducing the chance of discomfort or pain. The better penetration feels, the easier it is for both of you to relax and enjoy the experience. Lube also makes long anal play sessions possible. No matter how small or large the finger, cock, or toy, *you need lube*.

There are many different varieties of lubricants on the market, with the widest selections at sex toy shops and websites. Many of these places carry small sample sizes or a sampler pack, which is ideal; it's best to experiment with different brands to see what's right for you.

Oil- or Vegetable-Based Lube

It's no secret that some people look no further than their kitchen or bathroom to find a lube. People write to me all the time and tell me that they use common household items—like olive oil, baby oil, Crisco, Vaseline, or lotion—as lube. They weren't made for bedroom activities so they definitely don't work as well as the many lubricants on the market which are formulated, tested, and designed specifically for sex. There are lubricants sold that have similar properties, brands like Boy Butter, Elbow Grease, and ID Cream. These lubes are slick and greasy, often with a creamy consistency reminiscent of Crisco. They are great for male masturbation, and although they are marketed for anal sex (especially toward the gay male consumer), the problem with them is the same as with household products: they are oil based or vegetable based. This group of lubricants breaks down latex condoms, dams, and gloves, so you should use them with latex alternatives like vinyl or nitrile. They often stain sheets, clothing, and towels, and are generally hard to clean up. In addition to being incompatible with latex, oil- and vegetable-based lubes can wreak havoc on a woman's pussy. Even when you're headed for her ass, and you are being diligent about ass to pussy cross-contamination, sometimes a little lube finds its way into her front door. In this case, that lube cannot be rinsed out, is a perfect breeding ground for bacteria, and will most likely cause an infection of some kind. For all these reasons, I do not recommend oil or vegetable-based lubes for anal play.

Desensitizing Lube

With popular brand names like Anal Ease, Anal-Eze, and Tushy Tamer, "desensitizing" lubes promise to make anal sex easier and more comfortable. Don't believe the hype! These lubes contain benzocaine (or a similar ingredient), a topical anesthetic that numbs your anus and rectum. It's the same ingredient in "delay" or "prolong" creams to help men maintain an erection longer. I absolutely do not recommend using these products or others like them, ever. Because they have the effect of numbing your anal area, you literally cannot feel your ass and you are in danger of hurting yourself. Plus, some people are allergic to benzocaine.

Anal sex should never, ever be painful. If it hurts, stop. Pain is your body's way of telling you that whatever you're doing isn't working. You should always listen to your body. Using desensitizing lubes can lead people to go further than they normally would or take something bigger in their ass than they should. The result is a sore ass, possible tearing and damage to the delicate lining of the anal canal and rectum, and pain after the fact that isn't exactly going to make you want to rush right out and try anal sex again. Plus, on the off chance that the anal penetration is pleasurable, you won't be able to feel that either. A sticker on one of the bottles says it all: *Numbs your most sensitive parts*. Who wants that? They are a bad idea all the way around. Keep reading to learn about the many water-based and silicone lubricants that are great for anal penetration.

Water-Based Lube

Water-based lubes are nonirritating, nonstaining, odorless, and easy to wash off toys and bodies. They either have no taste or a faint taste. Thin, liquidy lubes are very popular for vaginal penetration because they have a similar consistency to natural vaginal secretions. Popular brands include Aqua Lube, Astroglide, K-Y Liquid, Probe Silky Light, and Wet Light. While these slick lubes can be somewhat effective for anal penetration, and will definitely do the job in a pinch, thicker water-based lubes are much better.

Thick water-based lubes have the same properties and advantages as their thinner counterparts, the only difference is in their consistency; they tend to feel more like hair gel or jelly. Many people like to use these thicker lubes for anal play because they provide extensive lubrication and tend to dry up less quickly than watery varieties. If they do dry up, add a little water or saliva to revive their powers. Their texture also means that they will coat and protect the delicate, sensitive lining of the anal canal and rectum. All water-based lubes are compatible with latex and nonlatex barriers as well as all sex toy materials.

Many people reach right for that tube of K-Y Jelly since it's one of the most recognizable and readily available brands. K-Y Jelly was designed for medical exams, which last only a few minutes, not for all-night sex-capades.[1] There are better thick lubricants out there with more staying power, including Astroglide Gel, Elbow Grease (Water-Based Formula), Embrace, ID Glide, K-Y Brand UltraGel, and Wet.

One unique lube which anal fans rave about is J-Lube. Originally designed as a veterinary obstetrics product for examining farm animals, vets use J-Lube to stick their hands up a cow to see if she's pregnant. It comes in a powdered form, which you mix with water, so you can control the consistency. Mixed with water it feels more like slime than liquid (and indeed special-effects designers often use it for its slimy properties); it coats your hand, glove, or toy in a unique way that makes it great for anal penetration, especially play with large toys or anal fisting. There is also a premixed formula (called J-Gel or Bear Lube) which is harder to find. Clean up with a little salt, since trying to wash it off with water will only make more lube!

Many women find that their vaginas can be sensitive or allergic to the most popular ingredient in water-based lube, the one that helps it stay wet: glycerin. Anecdotally, there seem to be more reactions to lubes with glycerin with vaginal penetration than anal penetration. If you or your partner is sensitive or allergic to glycerin, you may want to try a lube with vegetable glycerin (which discourages yeast growth) like O'My or Probe Thick and Rich or a glycerin-free lube. Because glycerin-free lubes dry up quicker than lubes that contain glycerin, they may be less ideal for anal play. Popular brands like HydraSmooth, Liquid Silk, and Sensual Power may be too thin and liquidy to do the job, so try thicker brands like Maximus, Sensua Organics, or Slippery Stuff Gel. Flavored lubes are also safe for anal penetration.

Good Anal Lubes

WATER-BASED: Astroglide Gel, Elbow Grease (Water-Based Formula), Embrace, ID Glide, J-Lube, K-Y Brand UltraGel, O'My, Probe Thick and Rich, Wet

WATER-BASED & GLYCERIN-FREE: Maximus, Sensua Organics, Slippery Stuff Gel

SILICONE: Eros Gel, Eros Power Cream, ID Millennium, Wet Platinum

Ask the Anal Advisor: *When Lube Comes Back Out*

Q: *I'm a heterosexual male. After about three years or so of trying, I've got my partner into anal sex. First, I worked her up into accepting two fingers, then I worked her up to my cock. As suggested I used lots of lube, the thick stuff; I also ejaculated in her ass. Later that day she complained of having really loose stool and a watery discharge. Could this be from her body expelling an abundance of come or using too much lube? I love ass play but I don't like the idea of wrecking someone's plumbing for the day. What's the best way of lubing someone without overdoing it?*

A: Many people experience runny or loose bowel movements after extended anal play, so your girlfriend's experience is a common one. Unfortunately, what goes in must come out, and while some of the water-based lube will dry up and some will be absorbed into the body, the rest has to get flushed out of the rectum the old-fashioned way. Plus, most water-based lubes contain some form of glycerin (which helps lube stay wet), and glycerin is used in suppository form for constipation, so—well, you get the idea. You may want to try a glycerin-free lube, like Maximus or Slippery Stuff for example, or one with glycerin low on the list of ingredients. Another alternative is to experiment with silicone lubes. Silicone stays wet much longer, and so you need a fraction of the amount you'd use in a water-based lube for penetration. Eros makes a silicone gel version which I definitely recommend.

The newest lubes on the market are the warming lubes, water-based lubes that create a warming sensation when you use them. Popular brands include Astroglide Warming Liquid, ID Sensation, K-Y Warming Liquid and K-Y Warming UltraGel, Wet Warming Lubricant, and Sliquid Sizzle (a glycerin-free warming lube). Thus far, reports have been mixed: some people describe the effect as too subtle to be anything worth raving about. Others find the feeling too intense, almost like mild burning, which doesn't sound pleasant. Most warming lubes contain either honey or menthol to create the warming effect along with assorted chemical ingredients, all of which can irritate the sensitive tissue of both the front and back doors. While these are safe to use, keep in mind that everyone will react differently to the ingredients and to the effect. I recommend trying a sample to see if these lubes are right for you.

Silicone Lube

Most silicone lubes are slick and thin, which may not be ideal for anal pen-etration; some people really like the slick texture, while others feel *too much* friction, which can be uncomfortable. Eros makes two thicker ver-sions—Eros Gel and Power Cream—that are ideal for silicone and anal fans. While silicone lube does not get absorbed into the genital tissue the way water-based lube does, some women find that it irritates their deli-cate parts. Silicone can be harder to clean up since it is not water soluble, and not all soaps will dissolve it (I recommend using warm water and a liq-uid soap). Perhaps the biggest drawback is that they are incompatible with silicone sex toys. Silicone lube bonds to a silicone toy and ruins it forever. So, if you're a fan of both and want to use them together, make sure you cover all silicone toys with a condom first.

How to Use Lube

The rule of thumb when it comes to lube is "on, not in." In other words, you should pour lube *onto* whatever is going to be doing the penetration—a finger, a toy, a penis—rather than directly *into* any orifice. When it comes to anal penetration, there's no such thing as too much lube, and you should re-lube frequently. Keep a box of baby wipes nearby to control drips and for easy cleanup.

If you find that you have trouble getting the ass well-lubricated or you need extra lube for penetration with something of size, there are items on the market like the Lube Shooter and the Astroglide Shooter that solve this problem. The Lube Shooter is a disposable hard plastic syringe with a flared base that you fill with your desired lube (a process that can be a little messy). Insert the body of the syringe in the ass, push the plunger, and you've got lube right where you want it! Also disposable and easy to use, the Astroglide Shooter is a prefilled flexible rubber tube of lube with a long neck that can be inserted into the anal canal (after removing the tip, of course). Squeeze the tube, and lube goes into the ass. You can also fill up a plastic irrigation syringe (found at drugstores) or a stainless steel enema syringe (available at specialty stores) for the same purpose. (For more on these, see chapter 15 and the Resource Guide).

Ask the Anal Advisor: *Fucking a Fluid-Filled Bottom*

Q: *For the last few months, my lover had been hankering to try anal sex. After reading your advice, buying lots of lube, and experimenting with a host of toys, we finally managed to get his gorgeous cock all the way in my bottom and he fucked me—and I had a fantastic orgasm! Since he'd never had anal sex before, as you can imagine, he is now a very happy bunny and wants more! He currently has a fantasy about filling my bottom with lots of creamy liquid, and then fucking me like that. We've seen stuff like this in porn movies, but I'm curious about how they do it and how we should do it. What liquid do we use and how much would be safe? I've been giving myself brief enemas before our anal play so I'm kind of used to stuff being there. I'm not sure how long it'd stay there and if there are any safety concerns I should be aware of. Any suggestions?*

A: Thanks for sharing your fun fantasy with me and your fellow readers. In general, I am a purist about what people should put in their asses: I endorse only plain water, lube, ejaculate, fingers, cocks, tongues, and toys. I discourage exotic enema ingredients, ice cream sundae toppings, and other equally wacky substances. But, in the case of your sweetheart's idea, you're in luck. He can fill your ass with lube! There are several great water-based lubes on the market—including Hydra-Smooth, Sensual Power, and Liquid Silk—that have creamy consistencies. In fact, they have a look and feel that's a lot like a man's come (which I think may be what your guy is going for). Plus, they are lubricants, designed for penetration, and therefore totally safe! If he wants to really fill you up, you may want to buy a disposable plastic irrigation syringe (available at medical supply stores and some drugstores), which he can fill with lube, and "shoot" up your ass. If he succeeds in filling your ass, remember, what goes in must come out. You may be a little runny for a day, as all that lube works its way out of your ass, so keep that in mind; I'd avoid, say, silk pants for a few days.

You've got a lot of choices when it comes to lubes. As I said in the previous chapter, I do not recommend lubes that contain nonoxynol-9, which can aggravate both vaginal and anal tissue and increase the chances of STD transmission. Lube should feel good inside you; if your pussy or ass feels irritated or itchy or it burns or stings, you may be having a reaction to one or more ingredients in the lube you're using. The bottom line is: every lube formula is slightly different, so read the ingredients on the label carefully.

NOTE

1. From the K-Y site: "In controlled performance testing K-Y® Brand ULTRAGEL™ and K-Y® Brand Liquid Personal Lubricant are far superior lubricants, since they are smoother and last longer than K-Y® Brand Jelly." http://www.k-y.com/faq/index.jsp#Anchor5, May 22, 2005.

8

Anal Sex Toys

There are plenty of fabulous sex toys you can use to introduce yourself or a partner to anal pleasure or enhance your anal play. Many products are designed and marketed especially for anal sex, and others used for vaginal stimulation and penetration can also be used anally (see illustrations 9, 10, and 11). When choosing a toy, consider these questions:

What do you want the toy to do: should it vibrate, rotate, inflate?

What kind of sensation are you looking for: do you want something in your ass for a "full" feeling or do you want in-and-out fucking?

What do you want it to feel like: the softness of jelly rubber, the firmness of acrylic, somewhere in between?

What do you want it to look like: a rabbit, a cock, a nightstick?

How much do you want to spend: $10, $50, $200?

Anal Beads and Bead Toys

Anal beads are latex or hard plastic beads attached by a string (made of nylon or sometimes cotton) that runs through them, usually with a ring on the end. The beads are slightly bigger than marbles and can be even larger. The most popular beads are usually 1/2" in diameter. Because they are a cheaply made item, the plastic beads usually contain rough seams. Be careful of edges that feel sharp to the touch of the finger; you can file the edges down with a regular nail file or cover the entire string of beads with a larger-size condom. Condoms are a good idea anyway for anal beads, since nylon and cotton strings can be difficult to clean properly, and some people may

ASK THE ANAL ADVISOR: *Losing My Marbles*

Q: *In Anne Rice's erotic novel* The Claiming of Sleeping Beauty, *there is a scene where Beauty was made to play a game: Twenty roses were scattered all around a room where the Queen sat, and Beauty had to crawl around and pick the roses up and return them one by one to the Queen, all the while being flogged to keep up her pace. Every time Beauty would bring a rose, the Queen would stick a large gold marble in Beauty's ass. The trick being that the further along she got, the harder it was to keep going without dropping the marbles. My husband and I thought this was really hot, and we'd love to play it out, but we are concerned with the idea of losing a marble inside my ass. Could that happen, and if so, what could we do to prevent it? We have worked with anal beads before, but there are only so many on a string, and those knots can sting! What can you suggest?*

A: While I love erotic fiction as much as the next kinky reader, when it comes to representations of bondage, sadistic sensation play, and other BDSM activities, you need to remember that half of the stuff that fictional characters do in books isn't even physically possible, let alone safe or meant to be instructional. Many, but not all, writers of leather smut have never actually done any of the things they write about. Or, even if they are players in real life, often they still indulge in fantastic fantasies they know are great to jerk off to but they don't mean for anyone to try to replicate them. The scene you describe from *The Claiming of Sleeping Beauty* is an example of a sexy scenario that's not practical, and could be physically harmful.

In general, anything you put in the ass should have a flared base (like on a dildo or butt plug) or another way to stop it from going all the way inside (like the ring on the end of a string of anal beads). You should never put any find the knots in the string between beads feels uncomfortable inside the ass.

Because they can be poorly made and difficult to clean, anal beads are not always the safest toy. A better bet for bead lovers is a toy based on the bead concept, made without string, as one continuous piece. These are much easier to clean (specific cleaning tips are in the Sex Toy Materials section at the end of this chapter) and are generally a lot more

round objects—marbles, Super Balls, Ping-Pong balls, golf balls, ben wa balls, or any other kind of balls—in your rectum. Besides irritating your rectal tissue, they can also become irretrievable without a speedy trip to the emergency room. Only beads that are on a string or anal bead toys are safe for anal play. You've already played with anal beads, and you're right, most people find the knots of the nylon or cotton rope pretty uncomfortable. I have several suggestions for scenes that may appeal to you. If you want to be surprised, now is the time to stop reading and hand the book over to your husband. Several sex toy manufacturers sell toys that are a continuous series of beads, but the toy is all one piece (no string, no knots); some have several beads of the same size, while others have graduated beads that get larger and larger. Your husband can insert the first bead, send you off to retrieve rose #1, then slide the second bead inside, and so on. It creates a similar effect to the marbles with a toy that's completely safe. Or, if the goal is to make it increasingly difficult to keep the object inside your ass as you retrieve the roses, he can begin with a silicone butt plug, and with each new round, replace it with a plug made of a heavier material, moving from clear acrylic to glass to marble to stainless steel. I've used all of these high-end toys, and can tell you that when you stand up with a steel butt plug in your ass, it feels like a barbell that's fighting gravity! A similar effect can be achieved with only one butt plug and a series of small weights usually used for cock and ball play or genitorture. Find a way to attach the weights to the base of the plug (I suggest a small piece of string around the rounded base); you can keep increasing the amount of weight each time a rose is retrieved. Use the story in the book as inspiration, but then be creative and create a scene that's clever, cruel, or whatever works for you. Most important, make it safe.

comfortable. Bead toys can be made of jelly, rubber, or silicone and have anywhere from five to ten beads. In some toys, the beads are all the same size—from marble-size to the size of golf balls or even bigger— and in others, they graduate in size. For first timers, I recommend you pick small beads, and gradually work your way up to larger sizes if you discover you like them. Always choose a bead toy with a ring or base on the end of it.

For some people, the moment when the sphincter muscles relax and allow for that first pleasurable penetration is incredibly hot. Nina Hartley calls it "the pop," although, have no fear, there's no actual popping sound. For these folks, anal beads are perfect, since they can experience that initial penetration sensation over and over as the anus opens to accommodate the bead, then closes around it, then opens for the next bead, and so on. Insert one well-lubed bead at a time, giving the ass a chance to adjust to and relish the sensation of expanding then contracting around the ball. As the receptive partner, if you've been practicing your Kegel exercises, you will be more aware of these contractions and able to control them voluntarily. Many people like to insert the beads while having their genitals stimulated. Once they are all in (or as many are in as you want), you can (slowly!) pull the entire string of beads out, creating an entirely different, but equally intense, sensation. Some folks like this grand exit to happen when they feel close to orgasm, in order to push them over the edge; others like to wait until they are coming to intensify the climax. You can also keep them in until after you've come. Remember to withdraw the beads slowly and gently—pulling the entire string of beads out in one motion too quickly could be uncomfortable. As with any other toy, experiment and find out what works best for you.

Butt Plugs

"What's the big deal about a butt plug?" I get that question a lot, followed inevitably by: "It just plugs the butt? You mean it doesn't light up or spin while it's in there? It can't burn CDs or store data? It's not a two-way pager or a Play Station external device?" A butt plug does exactly what it sounds like it does. It's designed to slide into your ass and stay put. In our culture, people have grown so accustomed to everything having bells and whistles that a basic task-oriented sex toy baffles them. Sure there are dildos that glow in the dark, vibrators that masquerade as lipsticks, and battery-operated toys with twenty different settings. But sometimes less is more, and such is the case with the deceptively simple joy of a butt plug.

Designed with the butt in mind, butt plugs are usually narrowest at the top, thickest in the middle, and narrow just above the base, which is flared. The traditional shape of a butt plug looks like a teardrop with a thicker bottom, or a skinny pear; they can also resemble diamond or phallic shapes. Above the wide flared base, the plug's neck has the smallest circumference, designed to allow the sphincter muscles to close around it. Remember that we are all built slightly differently, so the ideal plug shape for one person may not work for another. For example, when I designed

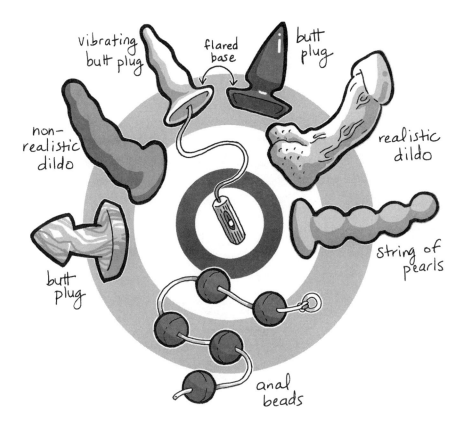

Illustration 9: Anal Toys

Ask the Anal Advisor: *Vegetables*

Q: *I'm twenty-nine years old, and I have been putting things up my ass for about ten years now. I've worked my way up to take the equivalent of three cucumbers. The last time I put things up my ass, the most bizarre thing happened, and it happened once before about a year ago. I like watery vegetables because I feel like I need less lube and my ass gets a "wet silk" feeling from them. After I inserted a peeled cucumber, I had this allergic reaction all over my body. The same thing happened last year with a carrot. Nothing grave, just red, itchy skin and swollen eyes, et cetera, which went away in about an hour. I know what it is since I've been allergic to lots of stuff since I was a child and still have serious hay fever. Is it the absorption of the vegetable juices by my rectum that causes the allergy or something else?*

A: There is a reason that household objects are household objects; they each have a purpose, and it's not sexual. I am thrilled that you've discovered anal penetration as part of your masturbation ritual, but I really don't want to encourage you to grab the hairbrush, the shampoo bottle, the cucumber, or anything else lying around. Has it been done? Of course, but I don't condone it. Of all food allergies, allergies to vegetables are not as common as others, however there is some research that shows that certain foods—including melon, banana, zucchini, and cucumber—as well as the popular herb chamomile, can aggravate ragweed allergies. Symptoms include itching and tingling of the mouth, lips, throat, and ears, and in more serious cases, the swelling of tissue or anaphylactic shock. You said that you have allergies and hay fever, so my guess is that you're allergic to ragweed, and some of the vegetables you're sticking up your ass are exacerbating this allergy. I really recommend that you buy a dildo. You need something with a flared base for anal penetration; it's an absolute necessity, so the object doesn't get sucked into your ass or lost somewhere in your rectum. Sex toys were manufactured with sex in mind, they are designed for penetration, and therefore much more ideal for it than a makeshift dong. There are relatively inexpensive dildos on the market, especially the rubber or jelly variety (silicone dicks are much more expensive). Buy yourself a fifteen- or twenty-dollar dildo, and I promise it will be well worth the investment.

the Tristan plug with Vixen Creations, we created a shape that would go in and stay in, especially if you wanted to keep it in for a while. It was designed for the widest part of the plug to slip just past the sphincter muscles so the plug would rest snuggly inside. A friend of mine tried it, and told me that rather than doing that, in her ass, it seemed to rest right at the sphincter muscle, which was very uncomfortable. Her internal geography just was not compatible with the toy's shape.

Butt plugs may be smooth or textured with ridges, ripples, rings, or bumps. The textures provide extra stimulation to the nerve endings in the area, especially as the toy goes in or comes out. Some butt plugs vibrate, others don't; beginners may find a vibrating butt plug a good choice since the vibration not only feels good but also helps relax the sphincter muscles. Plugs may be made of flexible materials like rubber and silicone or solid ones like clear acrylic, glass, or metal. They come in a whole bunch of sizes, and remember that it is always best to start small and work your way up. From the shape of a slim tapered finger to the size of a wide traffic cone, the diverse butt plugs in the world represent our collective imagination, fantasies, goals, and desires.

If you like the feeling of something just being in your ass, and appreciate the fullness and pressure without necessarily any moving in and out, then you would probably love a butt plug. Butt plugs are meant to go in and stay in. No need for lots of in-and-out play, just the sensation of the sphincters closed around the base of a butt plug, and you're in heaven. Once you slowly slide a well-lubed plug inside the ass, you can then move on to something else—clitoral stimulation, a blow job, vaginal penetration, whatever you'd like—and the butt plug will continue to stimulate without a lot of work on your part. If your partner loves having her nipples sucked while her ass is fucked, or if you want to concentrate on sucking his penis and he wants something up his butt, you could feel like you're playing Twister. A butt plug is a great solution!

Butt plugs are also a great way to warm up the ass for bigger things to come. Putting in a plug and leaving it in for a while lets the ass get used to having something inside it. Using a series of different sizes of plugs can help you work up to having something larger in your ass, like a dildo or penis. Butt plugs work while you play: the ass gets further aroused, relaxes, and opens up, all thanks to the plug. When you slip it out, the ass says, "Bring it on!" (i.e., it's ready for something bigger).

I have a clear acrylic butt plug (designed by Ray Cirino at Innerspace) that acts as a magnifying glass once it gets inside. It's a definite crowd-pleaser at workshops. Have you ever looked all the way inside someone's ass? I have and whoever I peer into, his or her ass is always clean, pink, happy, and healthy—truly a wonder to behold. Sex activist Annie Sprinkle once closed her one-woman show by slipping a speculum inside her pussy and showing audiences her cervix. It was a bold, educational, revolutionary display of female sexual power, and I pay homage to her each time I reveal someone's ass with my see-through plug. Armed with a flashlight (so geeky, I know), I shine some brightness on a part of the body we often don't see so intimately. It gives new meaning to being able to see what you are doing.

Some people like to wear a butt plug for a more extended period of time or even outside the comfort of their bedroom or home. For more information on wearing a butt plug long term, see chapter 14.

If you have a butt plug in, you may find that when you get really aroused or during orgasm, the plug inadvertently slips (or even shoots!) right out of your ass. While this may be surprising or embarrassing, don't be alarmed, it's pretty common. Remember that during arousal, your genital muscles contract, and those contractions may actually push a plug out of your ass. This doesn't necessarily mean that the plug is too small and you need to run out and upgrade—it's just a signal that you were very turned on!

Anal Probes and Vibrating Toys

For people who like stimulation of those fabulous nerve endings in the anal area, vibrators deliver consistent and powerful sensations; vibrating toys also help relax muscles, making them a great choice for anal play. Beginners may want to try an anal probe, which is a long, slim toy made of flexible rubber that vibrates; some also bend so you can customize the probe to hit just the right spot. If it bends or has a curved shape, you want to aim the curve toward the front of the body to stimulate the G-spot or the prostate. If you're a fan of dual action vibrators (like the popular Rabbit Pearl), there is one that has a small attachment the width of a small finger that is great for anal novices. There are also various attachments and sleeves that fit on standard-size vibrators or vibrating eggs to transform them into anal penetration toys. There are even remote-controlled vibrating butt plugs for people willing to give the power over to someone else.

If you're going to put a vibrator in your ass, it must have a flared base or be attached to a battery pack; this is especially important for vibrators since many of them are designed for vaginal penetration and don't have a base. If you already own a silicone toy like a plug or dildo and want to make it a vibrating toy, you can use any kind of vibrator to do so. Simply press a vibrator against the base of the toy once it's inside someone's ass, and the silicone conducts that vibration from end to end.

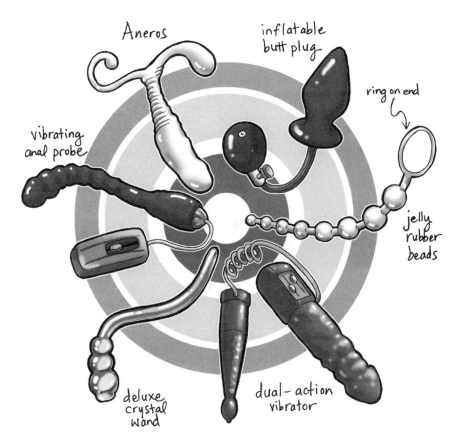

Illustration 10: More Anal Toys

Dildos

Dildos come in so many different shapes and sizes that there is one for practically every individual taste, need, and desire. Your first consideration should be an aesthetic one: are you into shades of skin color or are you more of a sparkles and swirls kind of girl? There are dildos that look like penises (with balls and realistic-looking heads), dildos that look like torpedoes, and even dildos that look like dolphins. Like butt plugs, they come with different textures as well as different degrees of firmness. Dildos can be made of nearly every sex toy material from flexible rubber and silicone to solid acrylic and glass. They can range in size from that of a fat magic marker to a 13" long phallus—and bigger. Dildos that curve up from the base (instead of being straight) are well suited to anal intercourse because they nicely mirror the curve of the rectum and you can stimulate the G-spot or prostate with them. Dildos are the best tools for in-and-out penetration. You can use a dildo with or without a partner. With a partner, a dildo can be just the thing you need to satisfy the craving to fuck and be fucked. It can also be used as a warm up tool for your ass, before a larger dildo or penis. Some people like to penetrate their partner with a dildo held in their hand; this tends to give the active partner more control of the dildo and its movement. Others like to strap a dildo to their bodies for an altogether different adventure.

Strap-on Dildos and Harnesses

If you want to have a hands-free fuck or your partner craves being fucked in the ass with a cock, strap a dildo between your legs and satisfy those desires. With a strap-on, a woman can put her whole body behind the penetration, and feel what it's like to shoot from the hip, so to speak. People also like the closeness (of body and mind) that a strap-on affords partners during penetration. I recommend a slim dildo (about 7 inches long) and a simple, functional harness of your choice.

There is a growing selection of harnesses made of leather, vinyl, nylon webbing, and even denim; two of the best manufacturers of quality harnesses (who also do retail sales) are Stormy Leather in San Francisco and Aslan Leather in Toronto, Canada. Your choice of material depends on how you want your harness to look and how much money you want to spend.

Ask the Anal Advisor: *Ejaculating Toys*

Q: *I have a question about ejaculating dildos and butt plugs. I saw a "recipe" for come that is made up of condensed milk, egg white, and sugar. Or what about just plain milk? I want to use an ejaculating dildo and actually make it ejaculate in my ass. Is it safe to use this "come" in my ass? Could this cause any medical problems?*

A: Ejaculating dildos and butt plugs are lots of fun; they give you the opportunity to experience shooting a hot load up your own ass or the rear of a friend. My first experience with a squirting dong came when I was sucking off a butch girl; she slammed her cock into my mouth, and at the same time squeezed her balls. Suddenly, a burst of fluid shot to the back of my throat, and the surprise alone made me soak the wood floor I was kneeling on!

I've heard that different people swear by different formulas for the perfect confection of fake jizz. The one that you describe (made of condensed milk, egg white, and sugar) creates an impressively lifelike texture and aesthetic; if you were going for great visuals—a pop shot on someone's mouth or tits, for example—that recipe would work well. If, however, your come shot is meant to be an internal one, then I've got two concerns when it comes to these confections. Because the rectum absorbs things quickly and easily, a shot of sweet faux come could leave you with a stomach ache. It is also a bitch to clean out of an ejaculating toy. For these reasons, I recommend two alternatives: use a creamy lube like Hydra-Smooth, Liquid Silk, or Sensual Power, which all have the look and feel of ejaculate. Or just use plain warm water, which still feels pretty real inside your ass.

Harnesses come in several styles, and your selection should depend on both function and aesthetics (see illustration 11). They all have an adjustable strap that goes around your hips. There is a basic triangle harness with one strap that fits between your legs; this harness tends to fit especially petite women the best. Because it fits like a G-string, the center strap rubs against your genitals, which may feel stimulating to some and annoying to others. There is a two-strapped harness with a triangle front that you wear like a jockstrap; this style places the straps around your asscheeks, leaving your vagina and ass easily accessible and free to be stimulated. People find that the two-strap harness tends to give them more control than the one-strap model; the dildo moves around less and is easier to guide. Both of these triangle styles have a hole where you slip the dildo through, resting it against your pubic mound.

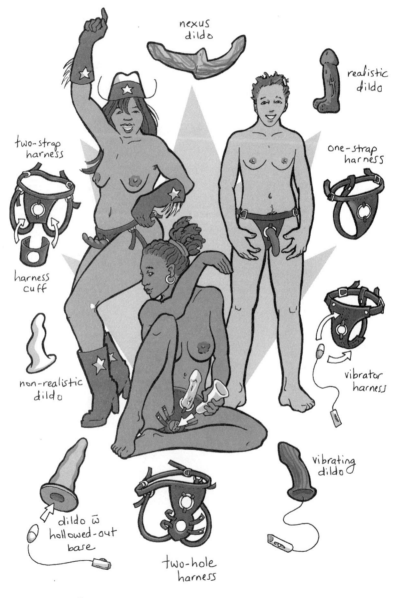

nexus dildo

realistic dildo

two-strap harness

one-strap harness

harness cuff

non-realistic dildo

vibrator harness

dildo w̄ hollowed-out base

two-hole harness

vibrating dildo

Illustration 11: Strap-on Dildos and Harnesses

If you prefer something between you and the dildo, there is a two-strap harness with a piece of material behind the cock ring. This style (sometimes called the Terra Firma harness) also allows you to change the size of the cock ring, which is especially good if the dildo you are using is significantly smaller or larger than an average-size one. You also have a choice of fasteners on your harness, either buckles or D-rings. There are plenty of other styles, including those made to fit plus-size women. See what fits you best and is easiest for you to adjust.

You want to choose a harness that fits you well—the snugger and more secure the better. I recommend that you try a few different styles on before you buy them or if you order from a catalog, see what the return policy is. The majority of dildos will fit in a standard harness, as long as there is a flared base and the dildo isn't excessively large. For beginning anal players, I would recommend a smaller dildo to start out.

For some women, when the base of the dildo rubs against the clitoris and vagina, there is enough friction there to feel fantastic. You should also consider the power of having balls. Some women simply don't choose a dildo with balls because they prefer a more nonrealistic-style dildo; however, balls do more than make it look real, they extend the base of the dildo and cover more surface area—which means more for you to rub up against. Think about it. If you want to add a vibrator to the equation, you've got several options. You can select a vibrating dildo, which will deliver vibration to you and your partner. You could try to don a wearable vibrator beneath the harness, but this may be awkward and interfere with the harness being tight enough. A better idea is the Buzz Me harness made by Stormy Leather and equipped with a pocket for a small vibrating egg. There are also dildos with hollowed-out bases made for vibrating eggs; choose a small vibrator or one more powerful with a battery pack; tuck the battery pack in the side of the harness and you're ready for vibrating action! For double penetration (one for you, one for your partner), there are harnesses with two holes, one for the dildo to penetrate you with, another for a dildo pointing in your partner's direction. The Nexus by Vixen is not an extra-long jelly dong like you see in adult novelty stores. Instead, it's a two-dildos-in-one package: the harness wearer can have a dildo inside her pussy or ass while simultaneously penetrating her partner. I just love sex toy technology! (For more on strap-on anal sex, see chapter 11; for more on male anal pleasure, see chapter 12).

Inflatable Toys

Inflatable butt plugs may look like bachelor-party gag gifts, but they are sex toys that actually work. Some of my best friends swear by inflatable plugs! One selling point is that you can gradually work your way up from slim to sizable without having to buy four different size butt plugs. You can track your progress, and one toy can suit your different desires. Other people like to feel something expand inside them. Once the plug is inside you, you can give your ass time to relax, then one pump, and you feel more full. Like with all kinds of anal play, don't try to rush things—take your time. Use common sense and never overinflate one of these bad boys. Make sure you first inflate it outside the body, and note how many squeezes of the inflating pump it can take, since you don't want to find out its limit while it's up your butt. According to all the letters I receive, and the people I meet at my anal sex workshops across the country, I know of only two people who've ever experienced an inflatable plug bursting. Both times, it wasn't a manufacturing defect, but the user's overzealousness.

Anal Toy Tips

CLEAN: Anything you plan to put in an ass—fingers, toys, a penis—should be clean. Because each sex toy material is different, follow the care and cleaning recommendations in the next section. Never submerge a vibrating toy in water unless it's waterproof. Alternatively (or in addition), you can cover a toy with a condom.

SMOOTH: Never put any sharp object or anything with rough or jagged edges in the rectum. *Never* put anything breakable in the ass.

LUBRICATED: No matter what the size, shape, texture, or material of a toy, always use plenty of lube, and be sure to use the appropriate kind of lube (remember, no silicone lube on silicone toys).

WARMED UP: Any toy that's bigger than a finger is not a starter toy. Begin with fingers or a slim toy to warm up the ass before putting a bigger toy in it.

FLARED BASE: Whatever kind of toy you select, it must have one important feature: a flared base. Perhaps you have heard rumors about people "losing" objects in their rectums and rushing to the emergency room. Or maybe you've seen one of several websites that document with X-rays the different items people have put in their rectums. While part of this is pure urban legend, the truth is you can get something lost in your ass if you aren't careful. Once you are aroused, your pelvic muscles contract, and this could cause your ass to suck something all the way inside it; then, your sphincter muscles close and it's stuck. A flared base prevents a toy from going beyond the rectum and is the best way to prevent your own trip to the ER.

REALISTIC SIZE: It's not a good idea to put something of an unrealistic width, length, shape, or size in someone else's or your own ass. Be sensible.

Sex Toy Materials, Care, and Cleaning

Rubber and Jelly Rubber

The most popular sex toy material is latex rubber. Rubber toys are relatively inexpensive, widely available, and come in a wide variety of sizes, shapes, colors, and textures. A majority of realistic-looking dildos, dual-action vibrators, and inflatable toys are rubber. They are a great choice for sex toy beginners, since you can try out different ones without breaking the bank. Rubber toys are compatible with water-based and silicone-based lubricants, but not oil-based lube. Made of a different type of rubber, jelly toys have a clear, jellylike appearance and tend to be softer and more pliable than plain ol' rubber. Lots of people like jelly toys for their cool appearance and texture. You should only use water-based lubes with jelly rubber. Over the years, I've heard many complaints from women who have a bad reaction to a jelly toy; they've told me stories about how jelly toys can make their pussy itch, burn, or sting. Jelly toys are made of food-grade PVC with a softening agent added. Many contain phthalates, chemicals that help give them their squishy texture. Manufacturers of rubber baby and pet toys have stopped using phthalates because of their potential link to cancer, and some, but not all, toy companies have followed suit. For example, Vibratex (a maker of dual-action vibrators), Doc Johnson, and

California Exotics claim their toys are made without phthalates. Ask the retailer where you buy a toy, or look for *phthalates-free* on the label to make sure you're getting the highest quality jelly rubber available. Before you use a jelly toy, you should inspect it; if it has a strong odor or a chemical film on it, then it's past its prime and should be thrown away.

Rubber and jelly rubber are porous, which means bacteria can make its way into nooks and crannies and stay there, and these toys cannot be completely disinfected. If you plan on sharing a rubber or jelly toy, you should put a condom on it first. Clean rubber and jelly with a mild liquid soap or a sex toy cleaner and store it in a cool, dry place; never use dish-washing liquid or any cleaner that contains alcohol. If your sex toy cleaner contains nonoxynol-9 (which many do), make sure you rinse toys thoroughly so none of the chemical lingers on the toy. People who are sensitive or allergic to latex should not use rubber toys (or they should cover them with nonlatex condoms first).

CyberSkin and Thermal Plastics

Popular terms like CyberSkin, SoftSkin, and UltraSkin are all brand names for a form of thermal plastic, a material rumored to have been invented by NASA. Thermal plastic has made a big splash on the sex toy scene because it has an incredibly realistic look and feel; it's as close to skin as something synthetic has gotten. Some women are sensitive to this material (some thermal plastic toys contain latex, so those allergic to latex beware), and if you are, I recommend covering it with a condom. Use only water-based lube with these toys. They are very porous and more prone to nicks and tears, so handle them carefully. You have to clean a thermal plastic toy right after you use it. Wash it with mild liquid soap or sex toy cleaner, make sure it's completely dry, then lightly dust it with cornstarch. This last step is necessary in maintaining its unique, fleshlike texture. Store in a cool, dry place away from other toys.

Hard Plastic

Some vibrators and butt plugs are made of hard plastic. Because they aren't flexible, toys made of hard plastic should be used carefully in the delicate rectum. Hard plastic is nonporous, easy to clean, and conducts vibration well. Some less expensive toys made with this material have seams which may be uncomfortable for penetration.

Vinyl

If you've ever seen incredibly large dildos and plugs (especially at stores like Mr. S Leather), they are probably made of vinyl. Vinyl is less porous than rubber and jelly, slightly more durable, but still inexpensive. Vinyl toys are safe for people with latex allergies and safe to use with all types of lubricants; they can be washed with antibacterial soap and water. The same rules about sharing that apply to rubber toys apply to vinyl ones. Vinyl toys should be stored away from heat, light, and other types of toys.

Silicone

When it comes to pliable sex toy materials, silicone is top of the line. Silicone toys come in a variety of colors, shapes, sizes, and even textures; these toys have a smooth texture that isn't sticky like rubber can be, and, depending on the manufacturer, silicone can feel soft, firm, or very firm. In addition, it warms to the touch and conducts body heat and vibration. Silicone toys are completely nonporous, so they are easy to clean and disinfect. These toys are very resilient and last the longest of all flexible materials; silicone can tear, but it takes some pretty rough handling to do so. The only drawback for silicone toy lovers is that they cannot use silicone lubricants with them; in most cases, silicone lube bonds to a silicone toy and ruins it, so stick to water-based lubes. Silicone can be cleaned in a number of ways: wash with hot water and antibacterial soap; soak in sex toy cleaner; boil for about three minutes; or wash in the top rack of the dishwasher without detergent (which is too harsh for silicone). Store them in a cool, dry place, and keep them upright if possible to protect them from bending or breakage.

Acrylic

Toys made of acrylic are hypoallergenic, unique, beautiful, and expensive. Some acrylic toys that are less expensive contain seams, but top-notch acrylic toys are completely seamless. Even silicone, the smoothest of soft materials, has a little "drag" to it, whereas these toys create an amazingly smooth sensation for penetration. Lube clings to them nicely, too. Caring properly for acrylic toys is very important if you want to maintain their transparency and finish. They're nonporous, tough (nearly unbreakable), but they can be easy to scratch. Wash them with hot water and antibacterial soap or soak them in a diluted bleach solution (10 parts water, 1 part bleach), then rinse well. Don't boil them or run them through the dishwasher, and never use alcohol as it will ruin the material by causing tiny cracks throughout it. Dry acrylic thoroughly with a soft cloth and store toys in something soft, like a velvet or satin bag (which often comes with the toy).

Glass

Glass toys have properties similar to those of acrylic—crystal-clear beauty, seamless lube-friendly finish, hypoallergenic material—except, naturally, they have more weight to them. If a glass toy isn't made of Pyrex (the most common high-quality consumer brand), then it should be certified medical grade, temperature resistant, and chemical resistant; if you're not sure, ask the retailer before you buy it. Glass toys can be warmed up easily (so they conduct body heat well), but never boil or put in the dishwasher unless instructions say you can. Because they are nonporous, they can be washed with soap and water, soaked in diluted bleach, even cleaned with alcohol (unlike acrylic). Use common sense: if it chips or breaks, let it go to glass toy heaven.

Metal

For folks who like a smooth, firm, solid toy, metal toys offer a variety of styles as well as weights. They're durable, nonporous, and conduct hot and cold temperatures nicely. There are a variety of metal toys on the market, made of aluminum or stainless steel, and some are hollow while others are solid metal. Metal can be cleaned with hot water and antibacterial soap, diluted bleach, alcohol, or by being placed in the top rack of the dishwasher without detergent. Metal toys must be dried completely to prevent rusting. Store them away from light, and in their own soft bag or a sock, to protect them from other toys.

Sex toy makers have gotten very creative, and in addition to acrylic, glass, and metal toys, there are other one-of-a-kind creations that can be beautiful works of art in addition to orgasm-inducing erotic tools. I've played with polished granite anal plugs (from JT's Stockroom), handcrafted hardwood dildos and anal bead toys coated in nontoxic protective coating (from Toy Bag), an aluminum tuning fork toy (from Innerspace), and other fun, exciting gizmos. These out of the ordinary toys can create unique sensations, and just look really cool going in and out of your ass or a partner's ass; as a general rule, they are not for beginners. The most important thing is to read and follow all cleaning and care instructions carefully. The bottom line is you've got lots of choices. Take a trip to your local sex toy shop or adult video store, or go online to see what's out there and what you might like. See the Resource Guide at the end of this book for retailers throughout the United States and Canada that carry a full line of toys and sex supplies.

CHAPTER

9

Doing It for Yourself:
Anal Masturbation

Why You Should Masturbate

The best introduction to anal eroticism starts with your own behind. In the 1970s, consciousness-raising groups spawned by the women's movement encouraged women to explore their vaginas. They did gynecological self-exams with speculums to gain a better understanding of their bodies. The more knowledge women have about our own bodies, the more in touch we can be with our health as well as our sexual pleasure. But even the most enlightened among us are not as familiar with our asses as we are with our pussies. We are taught to think of them as private, dirty, and not a source of pleasure. Because of this, we may be alienated from a very important part of our own body, and masturbation can be a way to connect or reconnect, to literally and symbolically get in touch with our asses.

Unlike men, who only have to glance down to see one important source of their libidos, women have to find a well-lit room, a comfortable position, and a mirror just to see our own vaginas and clitorises. The same is true for our buttholes. Looking at your ass, touching it, stroking it, feeling how it responds to even the lightest touch can give you a world of information about anal eroticism. If you'd like to experience anal pleasure but you're skittish about first approaching it with a partner, self-exploration is a great place to start. Anal stimulation may at first be something you want to reserve for your "sex for one" occasions, which is

> *Be sweet to your little "rosebud."*
> —BETTY DODSON—

fine; there will be plenty of time to bring anal eroticism to sex with a partner when you're ready. Your own exploration can get your ass used to stimulation and penetration. Maybe you're unsure of how it will feel or how you'll respond to penetration. Beginning by yourself means that you can experience various sensations without the pressure of wanting to please your partner. You can take as much time as you need, go as slow as you want, make noise if you want, stop if you want, come if you want. You can experiment with various kinds of stimulation and try different toys to see what works for you. Remember, you are the key to your own sexual pleasure.

Masturbation of any kind can make you a better lover. Not only is anal masturbation fun, but through it you can learn more about what you like. Then, when you're ready to share it with a partner, you'll have information to communicate with him or her—information that will make the experience better for both of you. Experiencing anal pleasure by yourself can also help to reassure you that it *can* be pleasurable with a partner; you'll know what it feels like when it feels good.

I believe the best way to become skilled at doing something to someone else is to practice it on yourself first. If you want to penetrate someone else's ass, exploring your own anal area by yourself will give you insight into what's going on down there, including the ins and outs of the anus, anal canal, and rectum: the sensitive tissue, the all-important curves of the rectum, and the various sensations of anal stimulation and penetration. Self-pleasuring will also give you a good sense of what your partner might feel as you give him or her pleasure.

How to Masturbate

You may want to take a bath or a shower or give yourself an enema beforehand. The bath or shower will help you relax as well as give you an opportunity to get your butt nice and clean and ready for fun. Also make sure your hands are clean and your nails are trimmed neatly. Get a hand-held mirror and your favorite lube, and find a suitable private place. First, take some deep breaths for several minutes to relax. Perhaps you'll want to lie down on the bed, play some soothing music, or light some incense. These are simply suggestions—do whatever will relax *you*.

Ask the Anal Advisor: *Pumping*

Q: *My boyfriend and I recently discovered the pleasure of penis pumping, and I'm thinking of getting a clit pump. But lately I have been using my guy's penis pump on my asshole while I masturbate, and I love the sensation and the feeling. I was wondering if you have ever done this, and if it is a safe practice?*

A: Many men and women have discovered the joys of pumping. For readers who may not know about it, a penis pump works like this: Your cock goes inside a hard plastic cylinder which either has a built-in pump or an external one. As you pump, air is sucked out of the cylinder, and the vacuum-like suction sends blood rushing to the cock. This helps the cock become erect, enhances an erection by giving it a bigger appearance (temporarily), and creates a sucking sensation which many men love. Women can use the same pumping mechanism with a nipple attachment (a much smaller cylinder), which works great on the clitoris. There are also clit pumps on the market made especially for women. The same principles apply: blood rushes to the clit, making it more swollen (and often more sensitive) than usual. I've pumped my own clit, and find that not only is it hot to see my clit all fat and thick, but clitoral stimulation is a lot more intense after I've pumped. I've never used a pump on my butthole. The puckered skin of the asshole is sensitive tissue that's incredibly rich in nerve endings and gets engorged when you're aroused much like the rest of our genitals. So, it makes sense that when you apply suction to it, blood rushes to the area and creates a pleasurable sensation. Similar cautions for all pumping apply: use a little lube inside the cylinder for a comfortable, easier fit; be careful not to pinch the delicate skin when inserting it into the cylinder; do not over-pump or leave the cylinder on for too long.

Begin by masturbating as you usually do; start by doing what you know first, which for most of us will mean stimulating the vagina and clitoris. Bring out that favorite vibrator or dildo, turn on a hot porn video or a steamy movie—do whatever will get you aroused. Don't jump right into exploring your anus; instead, simply masturbate and get your entire body aroused.

Once you feel relaxed and ready to explore, find a comfortable position, one where you'll be able to stay for a while and where you'll have a good view of your butt. Lying on your back or sitting in a comfy chair or on the edge of the bed might be best at first so you can look in the mirror. Begin by looking at your anus. Just check it out—the shape, the size, the color. How does it look? Relaxed, tense, somewhere in between?

Chances are you've got some nervous energy, so begin with some relaxation techniques like deep breathing or meditation; you may also want to do some PC muscle exercises (see chapter 2) to get warmed up and get the blood flowing to your ass.

Gently massage your butt cheeks, inner thighs, and the area around your anus. Continue to massage, stroke, and explore the area, going at your own pace. Note how the opening responds to the massage around it. When you feel comfortable, lube up your finger and gently touch your anus. Make sure your finger is good and slippery. Don't penetrate it, just do some external touching. Stroke it, rub it, let the lube glide over your skin. Just stimulating the opening can be extremely pleasurable because of all the nerve endings in the area. You may also want to use a vibrator to stimulate the outside of your anus; vibrations can both relax the area and get the blood pumping there. Tune in to the sensations you feel, both in your anus and in the rest of your body. Keep touching, but just touching—no penetration of any kind yet. You can continue using the mirror, or put it down at any time. A good next step is to use your finger to press gently at the opening. Feel how your body responds to the pressure against it. Keep touching and pressing until you feel ready for more. You may want to continue to stimulate your clitoris to get further aroused; remember, masturbating gets the whole pelvic area stimulated and engorged.

If you want to explore penetration, begin with one well-lubed finger. You can also use a very slim sex toy. If you choose a toy, remember that it should have a flared base to prevent it from going too far into your ass. If you're using a dildo, it should have a base or be longer than 8" and have something to hold on to (like a baton-style dildo, which actually has a handle). I find that fingers are best to start with because you can really feel how your ass responds to stimulation, whereas with a toy, you may feel like you're flying blind. Plus, if the first finger that slips in your anus is your own, then someone else's won't seem so scary and may even feel better than you had imagined! Continue by adding more lube to your finger and inserting just the tip into your anus; stay there and let yourself get used to the feeling. Add some lubricant. Move your finger gently against the sides of the opening without going any farther inside. When you feel ready, venture a little farther. See how the sphincter muscles feel around your finger. You may want to continue to masturbate with your other hand or use a vibrator. Remember to be patient with yourself, go at your own pace, and listen to your body. If at any time you feel discomfort or pain, stop. There's no rush. Keep nudging the finger inside until it's as far as you want it to go.

Experiment with all the different sensations you can create with just one finger. You can try a slow probe, venturing inside inch by inch, experimenting with a variety of depths. Some people like a circular motion, creating circles just inside the anus with a finger and feeling the walls of the anus contracting around the finger. Other people enjoy the feeling of simply having something in their ass; see what it feels like to rub your clitoris while your finger stays still in your ass. You can also practice some in-and-out play, trying different speeds and rhythms as you slide your finger in and out of your anus. Savor each new movement and sensation.

As you become more experienced, you can repeat this exercise with more lube and more fingers. When you can comfortably fit about two fingers inside, you may want to graduate to a butt plug, dildo, or vibrator. Remember, plugs are good for that full feeling, dildos for in-and-out action, and vibrators for in-and-out and, of course, vibration. Because these toys are longer than your fingers, you can use them to probe more deeply into the rectum. Make sure to use plenty of lube and start out slowly. Pay attention to how the muscles contract around the toy; make sure to let your ass get used to the feeling each time you inch a little farther inside. You'll notice a difference as your tool moves from the anal canal into the rectum. In the anal canal, you'll experience more resistance and a tighter feeling. In the rectum, you will feel like there's more room. If you rush penetration, your anus is likely to get sore and you'll have to stop all activities before you might want to. If you listen to your body and give yourself a chance to get fully aroused, your ass will open up and give you plenty of room for penetration by a slim dildo and, eventually, even bigger things, if you want.

QUOTE

Betty Dodson, *Sex for One: The Joy of Selfloving* (New York: Three Rivers Press, 1996).

10

Let Your Tongue Do the Walking:
Analingus

Analingus, known more commonly as "rimming," is stimulation of the anal area with the mouth and tongue—licking, flicking, nibbling, sucking, circling, and tongue-fucking. Many people love the simple pleasure of having their ass licked or licking a partner's ass. Because the anal area is so full of nerve endings, even the tiniest sensations can register high on the turn-on meter.

Hygiene

Lots of people feel especially anxious about rimming because of the association between the anus and defecating; we learn at an early age that if something is dirty or smells bad, we shouldn't put it in our mouth—or put our mouth on it. Remember that there are normally only trace amounts of feces in the anal canal and if the receiver has bathed beforehand, there won't be any around the external opening. If you and your partner are especially concerned about cleanliness, your partner could have an enema. (Remember an enema should be done at least two hours before the sexual encounter). Analingus need not be any more dirty or messy

Ask the Anal Advisor: *My Ass Licking Hang-Up*

Q: *My girlfriend wants me to kiss and lick her anus. I find this difficult to do because I was raised by strict Catholic parents who taught me that shit is dirty. I sniffed her asshole and it did not smell. I also licked all around it, but I could not bring my tongue to her little rosebud. I kept imagining it opening up and shit coming out of it. But when my girlfriend licked my anus, I ejaculated uncontrollably onto her chest. It felt great! How can I get past my hang-up?*

A: It's not just God-fearing Catholics who shy away from ass-to-mouth action; actually, plenty of folks have a fear of shit that prevents them from exploring many different forms of backdoor love, including being tongue-tied inside a sweetie's ass. Empty bowels and a hot soapy shower will ensure that your anal romp with your partner will be nothing but good clean fun. However, if you are especially concerned about cleanliness—and judging by those powerful poop images you are having, I'd say you are—then you may want to ask your girlfriend to have an enema before you go anywhere with that reluctant-yet-potentially-eager tongue of yours. You may also want to consider using a dental dam or some plastic wrap as a barrier between your mouth and her butthole. Since you have obviously experienced the ecstatic pleasures of rimming from the other end, you owe it to yourself and your girlfriend to give it right back to her. Sexual double standards suck, and it's not fair that you should be sitting on her face without letting her sit on yours.

than cunnilingus. Some people find the anus disgusting or gross, just as some unenlightened folks find the vagina and clitoris unappealing. Yet many of us approach cunnilingus with desire and enthusiasm and feel the same about analingus.

Analingus Tips and Techniques

A good way to introduce rimming is to begin nibbling and licking your partner's asscheeks. As is true for other activities, it's important to explore and pleasure the whole area, rather than diving right into the crown jewel.

I trace my tongue up and down her crack, so gently, full of hot breath, I want her to feel the heat even through the barrier, want her to be able to imagine it isn't there. I start to work my tongue in a little deeper, wriggling it against the sensitive spots, taking long, long licks from just below the opening of her cunt over and past her asshole, licking a fraction harder with each swipe of my tongue. She sighs, shifts her hips, presses against me. Encouraged, I keep on, starting to vary the pressure and depth of each lick, sometimes using the broad flat of my tongue and sometimes just the very tip, as hard as I can make it; I trace around the opening of her asshole, crinkled tightly shut, tracing my tongue along each of the tiny sunburst furrows of skin that radiate out from it, trying to get it to trust me.

—S. BEAR BERGMAN—

Once you're ready to put your mouth on the anus, start out slowly. Let your mouth, lips, and tongue explore freely, and experiment with different techniques as you go along. Listen to your partner's verbal and nonverbal responses and let those help guide you. Brush your lips against the opening, letting your bottom lip drag and linger there. Lick around the opening making a circular motion with your tongue. Start at the pucker and move out toward the cheeks, repeating this technique all the way around. Reverse this motion: begin at the outer edge and move toward the center. Let your tongue slip into the hole gently, then back out. Try thrusting your tongue in and out, penetrating your partner's ass.

There are a variety of positions you can try for analingus. Some people like to lick their partner's anus from behind in the doggie-style position, with the receiving partner on hands and knees. Others like to create a version of the sixty-nine position, so they can pleasure each other simultaneously. You can lick your partner's anus from almost any position, including standing, sitting, or lying down. Experiment with what is most comfortable and pleasurable for both of you.

Rimming can be incredibly pleasurable for everyone involved, including the person giving the pleasure. Nina Hartley demonstrates in her anal sex video: "Rimming is extremely, extremely pleasurable... It's important to keep in mind that if you're performing analingus, give your mouth a good time. Again, it's never something that you're just doing to the other

---

Ask the Anal Advisor: *Cotton Mouth*

Q: *I am a newcomer to analingus, and I've only performed it on my girlfriend a few of times. Every time I do, my mouth gets extremely dry. Why is that?*

A: As an avid ass-eater myself, I've never run into the problem you describe. But that doesn't mean it's not possible. There is nothing inherent to rimming that leads to a dry mouth, but there are a few possible explanations for your condition. As you lick your lover's butthole and spread your saliva around, you may be sharing more spit than your mouth is producing, leading to an imbalance. You may also be dehydrated, which is easily rectified by drinking plenty of fluids before you dive back in. If it's still uncomfortable, then I suggest you rub a small amount of lube (either a flavored one or one with a taste you don't mind) on her pucker before you kiss it. Your dry mouth is most likely unrelated to your ass licking altogether: many medications can cause a dehydrated mouth, as can common substances like tobacco, alcohol, and caffeine. If this parched condition persists, you should see your doctor.

---

person; it's something you're sharing with each other. As happy as my [ass] is, his mouth is equally as happy."[1]

You can combine rimming with other oral pleasure. During a blow job, tease his balls with your tongue, then move down to his ass. Or, after licking your partner's pussy, let your finger take over for your mouth to stimulate her, and venture to her ass to give it some oral attention.

Analingus and Safer Sex

One of the golden rules of anal play is that if something goes in an ass, it should never be inserted in a pussy without a thorough washing or a new condom, glove, or dam. Does that mean you can never go from analingus to cunnilingus without spreading germs? The reason that going directly from ass to pussy is not a good idea is because you can introduce bacteria from the rectum into the vagina, where it will cause an infection. There is a much greater risk of this transfer of bacteria during penetration because a finger, cock, or toy has been inside the rectum (the deeper you go, the more likely you will come into contact with bacteria or trace amounts of fecal matter). When it comes to oral stimulation, if you are simply licking the outside or just inside of your girlfriend's ass, then her outer lips and clitoris, there is less (but not zero) risk of cross-contamination, as long as her ass was clean to begin with. If you want to be super safe, you can rinse your mouth out with mouthwash in between oral acts or use separate dams for each activity.

If you plan to lick someone's ass, you should know the risks. You can be exposed to genital warts, genital herpes, chlamydia, gonorrhea, syphilis, and hepatitis A. If there are open sores on the anus or in the anal canal, you are at risk for hepatitis B, hepatitis C, and HIV. So you should practice safer sex by using an oral sex barrier like a dental dam, plastic wrap, an unlubricated condom cut lengthwise, or a latex glove cut into a usable shape. Dab some lube on the side of the barrier that covers the anus.

If you and your partner have tested negative for STDs and hepatitis and are in a monogamous relationship, licking ass is relatively safe. However, if you come into contact with any fecal matter, you can catch whatever is in the person's gastrointestinal tract, including parasites, worms, hepatitis A, and any other disease-causing organism living there. Normally, if someone has a gastrointestinal problem, he or she feels sick and is unlikely to be in the mood for ass licking. But it is possible to be infected and asymptomatic. As for E. coli, there is always some E. coli in the stool. If it's a disease-causing E. coli, then the person who has it is already sick and symptomatic, and you shouldn't lick his or her ass. If a person has no symptoms of E. coli disease, then you should be fine.

NOTE

1. Hartley, *Guide to Anal Sex.*

QUOTE

S. Bear Bergman, "Lessons," *Best Lesbian Erotica 2005,* edited by Tristan Taormino (San Francisco: Cleis Press, 2004), 128-129.

Anal Penetration

Beginning Penetration

Ready? Anal penetration is a huge subject, covering everything from penetration with fingers and small toys to a penis or strap-on dildo. Included here you'll find tips for both giver and receiver on communication, relaxation, warm-up, and positions, as well as techniques for strap-on sex and double penetration.

Make sure you have all the tools you want nearby—your favorite condoms, gloves, lube, toys, and baby wipes—so you don't have to go searching for them in the middle of a passionate moment. Review my recommendations about hygiene (chapter 4) and enemas (chapter 5), so your butt is prepared.

Take Your Time

The most common mistake people make—and the number one reason that the receptive partner ends up in pain—is that they rush penetration. In a typical straight adult video, a guy with an erection simply bends a

*He's moving in her, light and
quick, working her ass so sweetly
she wants to scream. She's going
to come. She stays there a while,
riding the knowledge, her clit full
and her cunt dripping and her ass
on fire. It's so dark with the
blindfold, and all she can think
about is how good it will be when
she comes, how good it will feel,
how it doesn't matter about her
ass being sore, how nothing
matters but this come.*
—ROSE WHITE AND ERIC ALBERT—

woman over and sticks his dick in her ass. People try the same thing at home with painful, sometimes disastrous results. In reality, on a porn set, women warm up with plenty of lube, fingers, and toys; the problem is that this foreplay ends up on the cutting room floor or never gets filmed in the first place. No one can go from zero to sixty in five seconds flat, not even the professionals.

If you've never done any anal play before and your goal is to have intercourse with a cock or strap-on dildo, or be penetrated by a large toy, *it's not going to happen in one night*. Anal penetration should be a slow, gradual process. Patience is crucial. Everyone must go at their own pace for anal sex to work. When both partners are patient, it's much easier to relax, especially for the receptive partner.

Because anal sex takes time, it's not a choice activity for a night when you just want a quickie, or someone has somewhere to be. If you are nervous, anxious, or stressed out about anal sex, sex in general, or the presentation you're giving tomorrow at work, anal sex should not be on the agenda. The more time you take in beginning, the more you'll benefit in the end.

Communicate

During a demonstration in one of my Anal Sex 101 classes, I was going to show some techniques on a woman I'd never played with before. We agreed that I would put a few fingers in her, then an acrylic butt plug. I asked her about what she liked and disliked, and if there was anything I should know before I put the plug in her ass. She responded, "Well, yeah. I want you to slide the plug in until you get to the widest part, then stop and let me get used to it. Tell me just before you're going to put it in further. Then, slide it all the way in. Once it's in, I will hate it and want you to take it completely out. Take it out, wait a minute, then you can slide it all the way back in." I asked her why she hated it, and she explained that the first time a plug fully penetrates her ass, the feeling is too overwhelming, and she needs it to stop immediately. But once she recovers from that, it can go back in and feel great. I loved how specific she was. I told her we'd follow her plan to the letter, but when the plug was all the way in the first time, I wanted her to say out loud, "I hate it!" which would be my signal to take it out.

She got on her hands and knees on a massage table. After warming up her ass with my fingers, I placed the plug at her anal opening and pressed slightly on the base to begin penetration, then I instructed her to push herself onto it. I told her to stop when she got to the widest part. We both took a deep breath.

"Ready?" I asked.

"Ready," she said. I continued my pressure on the base until it was at the widest part, then I stopped. When she said she was ready, I told her I was going to put the rest of the plug in her ass. I pushed gently on the toy and watched as it disappeared into her ass, until her sphincter muscles closed around the narrowest part just above the base.

"I hate it!" she screamed, and the audience laughed as I slid the entire plug back out. I squeezed some more lube onto the tip of the plug, and rubbed it around to distribute the clear gel. Then I proceeded to slide the plug back into her. As I got about halfway in, she said, "Wait, what are you doing now?"

"I'm putting it back in like you told me to."

"Oh, I was wrong. Give me a minute." The audience laughed again. I did too, because she was so adorable! We agreed that I'd play with her clit some more and just tease her opening with the toy. When she was ready, she told me, and I put the toy all the way in her ass. She moaned and said, "Yeah, that feels really good."

This is a good example of active communication and negotiation. As you begin anal exploration, tell each other how you're feeling, give and take instructions, communicate about what you need and want. Remember too that what you think your partner needs may change in the middle of it, so be prepared to be flexible.

Tips for the Receiver

Find a comfortable position. If you are a first timer, you may find that lying on your back works best since you can make eye contact with your partner, communicate face-to-face, and have your genitals easily accessible for stimulation. You may want to put a pillow under your butt to angle it for easier entry. Each person's body is unique, and what is a comfortable position for one may be uncomfortable for another. There's no rule about the greatest position for beginners, so explore to find what works for you and your partner. There will be a more in-depth discussion of positions later in this chapter.

RELAX

Relax, relax, relax. Take a deep breath. And another. Relaxation is so important to having pleasurable anal sex. With the hectic pace of our lives, it is one of the hardest states to achieve. Because the ass can be a place where we store much of our stress and tension, we need to give our bodies plenty of time to release that tension before venturing into anal pleasure. I find that doing about fifteen minutes of deep breathing helps my body to unwind, and the breathing actually gets me in touch with how my entire body is feeling. A warm bath, candles, and a sensuous massage are also great relaxers. We must also relax our minds, and some people like to meditate or do some positive visualization to calm and prepare themselves for anal penetration. Ultimately, our bodies and minds are linked, and we have the power to relax or to tense up.

Relaxation is also critical because anal penetration may feel strange at first. Some level of discomfort is common, especially for anal sex beginners. Our asses are used to pushing things out, not taking them in, so penetration is a new experience for them. Many people tell me they have the urge to have a bowel movement during anal sex; if that's the case for you, I recommend you stop and go to the bathroom. You may, in fact, have to go. But (since you already had a bowel movement to prepare) it's more likely that your body is just a little confused. Because the rectum is used to expelling things, when it feels something inside, it sends a signal to the brain to shit it out, which is what it normally does. The next time you feel like you have to have a bowel movement, I recommend you take several deep breaths, relax, and let your ass get used to whatever is inside it. Make sure that the finger or sex toy inside you stays put and doesn't make any sudden movements. Chances are after you relax, that initial feeling will subside, and you can progress to anal pleasure. Remember too that the more you practice anal penetration, the more your ass will get used to having things inside it, and will respond with less confusion and more pleasure.

When your partner first penetrates you, focus on relaxing the sphincter muscles. You may also want to bear down or push out to make penetration easier. It sounds like the opposite of what you're trying to achieve, but bearing down often helps the muscles to relax.

TAKE THE LEAD

Talk to your partner before, during, and after about what turns you on, the sensations you experience, what you'd like more of, and how everything feels. The more information you can give your partner, the better equipped he or she will be to please you.

You set the pace and control the action. I know it may seem like a contradiction—*I'm getting nailed in the ass, and I'm the one in the driver's seat?*—but you *are* the one calling the shots. You need to be well aware of your body, and specifically of your anal sphincters, because you have the ability to relax them. Listen to your body; if you feel any pain, you absolutely need to stop. Don't fool yourself that the pain will subside or pressure yourself to continue even when it no longer feels good. *Anal sex does not have to be painful at all.* I realize that there is a fine line sometimes between pain and discomfort, and each person is different. You need to judge for yourself where that line is. Give your partner plenty of feedback; tell him or her how slow or fast, how deep or shallow; if you want less or when you're ready for more. You must also be prepared to tell your partner to slow down, change activities, or stop altogether.

Tips for the Giver

TURN YOUR PARTNER ON

Start out with some fun, stress-free foreplay. One of the keys when trying something new is not to forget the tried and true techniques that are already working. Before you even go near your partner's ass, get him or her revved up in the usual ways—get things started with that favorite oral technique, position, sex toy, et cetera. Kiss her on that favorite spot of hers. Stroke that place you know will drive him wild. The more relaxed and turned on your partner is, the easier anal penetration will be. As you begin experimenting with anal stimulation and penetration, keep other kinds of stimulation going, whether it's hitting her G-spot, licking his perineum, or using a trusty vibrator.

As his mouth and tongue lapped at my tight, defensive buttyhole, the muscles gradually relaxed. By the time he gently pushed the head of his big oiled dick against my rosebud, I was so open and turned on that he eased inside with a minimum of discomfort. Then he slowly fucked me doggie style as I played with my clit. The orgasm was unforgettable.

—BETTY DODSON—

LISTEN AND TALK TO YOUR PARTNER

It's important that you focus on your partner as you're giving him or her anal pleasure. The receiver should feel comfortable to talk as much as he or she wants during the experience. Ask her how she feels; ask him what he wants. You should also listen to your partner's body. Feel how the sphincter muscles contract around your finger and respond to your touch. Observe the level of tightness and openness of the anus in addition to the rest of the body's response to anal stimulation. What verbal and nonverbal cues is she giving you? How is his breathing pattern? What kinds of sounds is she making? Tell your partner what you're doing, especially each time you are about to move on to something new. Also tell her or him what *you're* feeling, what's turning *you* on; it will enhance the communication and pleasure between you. Ask specific questions like: *How does this feel? Would you like more or less movement? Do you want me to play with your pussy while I'm doing your ass? Do you want more teasing? Some rimming? More pressure and fullness? Less in-and-out motion?* Ask.

Make sure your partner knows that if she wants you to stop, she need only say so and you will stop. Anal sex can be very highly charged even for the most willing, aroused, or experienced receivers. Having your ass penetrated can be intense, emotional, even a little scary. Keep all these factors in mind, and remember that your partner has put a tremendous amount of trust in you. Respect that trust as well as your partner's body. Realize that she or he may be feeling particularly vulnerable or may be a little anxious. Reassure your partner that she or he is in charge.

DON'T GO FROM ASS TO PUSSY

It can't be said too often: putting something in the ass and then transferring it directly to the vagina is a perfect route to a vaginal infection. Bacteria that lives naturally in the rectum (possibly along with some fecal matter) will be transferred to the pussy, and since the pussy doesn't naturally flush itself out, bacteria can set up shop, multiply, and live there until you treat it. Some women get yeast infections or urinary tract infections, others get bacterial infections like gardinerella.

Once anything—a finger, a toy, a penis—has been in the ass, it must be thoroughly washed or covered with a new condom or glove before it goes anywhere near the vagina. In addition, you should be aware that lube that goes into your ass and drips out of it can make its way to your pussy, which could also cause an infection. To prevent what I call "the drip-down effect," have a box of baby wipes handy to make a clean swipe of the area (always swipe front to back).

GETTING STARTED

When you're ready to introduce anal stimulation, start out by massaging the asscheeks and inner thighs. Work your way around the anal area with your fingers, your mouth, or a vibrator. Remember that the more you stimulate the entire area, the more the blood rushes there. You can combine anal stimulation with stimulation of the clitoris, vagina, or penis to get the entire genital region engorged and excited.

In the beginning, I like to start penetration with fingers rather than small toys since fingers are sensitive and connected to our brains whereas toys aren't. Putting your finger in someone's ass can give you a good idea of how that ass feels and responds.

When your partner is ready, use one well-lubed finger. Instead of going straight inside, touch the pad of your finger to the opening; this trick usually relaxes the anus, allowing you to slip your finger in comfortably. Go up to the first knuckle and just stay there. Since the first instinct of the sphincter muscles will be to tighten, let the ass get used to having something inside it and let the sphincter muscles relax. A good way to further relax the receptive partner's ass is to *slowly* and *gently* push up and down against the opening. Gently apply pressure downward toward the bottom of the anal opening; do the same thing upward, to the left, and to the right. I call this the North-South-East-West technique, and it's a simple, gentle way to let the ass know you're there. When your partner is ready for more, slip farther inside slowly and gently. Encourage him or her to breathe deeply; stay where you are on the inhale and nudge farther in on the exhale. Don't go too far too fast.

There are so many nerve endings in the anal area that every sensation is magnified. Keep in mind that a light touch, a slim pinkie, and a slight wiggle all go a long way. The simplest caress can be extremely pleasurable. In the beginning, it's best to err on the side of caution and gentleness. If your partner wants more, deeper, faster, or harder, he or she will tell you.

What If It Hurts?

THERE MAY BE TOO MUCH FRICTION. Withdraw, add some more lube, and see if it feels better.

Stop the movement of fingers, cocks, or toys, but stay inside; see if the pain subsides.

Decrease the number of fingers you have inside or use a smaller toy. Work your way back up, but never force anything.

Withdraw and focus on more external stimulation—a hand job, oral sex, more foreplay.

If you need to, stop the activity altogether. Allow your partner to relax, take some deep breaths, listen to his or her body.

WORK YOUR WAY UP

Once you have one finger inside your partner's ass comfortably, you can begin to experiment with different sensations. Stay still and stimulate his or her genitals, and see how the body responds. Move your finger in and out and explore different speeds. You can also try to make a twisting motion as you go in and out. Make sure that the receptive partner is the one in control of the action—and she should let you know if she wants more or less, slower or faster, deeper or not-so-deep. To get one finger in and bring your partner to orgasm is a good goal for an evening. I know it sounds like a small step, but the idea is to have a series of hot, pleasurable anal sessions to build on.

If you're both feeling ambitious and want more, slowly slide your finger out and add more lube. To go from one finger to two, cross your index finger over your middle finger, make sure both are well-lubed, and touch the pads of the fingers to the opening just like you did with one finger. Slide both fingers inside slowly, be still, and let the ass adjust. Remember your anatomy lesson and those two curves you're going to run into in the rectum. Each person's rectum is unique, so don't assume that a technique that worked on one person will make your current partner scream in ecstasy. Going slowly will help you navigate the curves of the rectum and begin to discover the individuality of your partner's anal canal and rectum without causing discomfort. There will be plenty of time later for a hard-and-fast frenzy, if that's what you both want. But, in general, you should-n't make any swift or jerky movements. Likewise, whenever you withdraw anything from the ass—if she asks you to stop, after she's had an orgasm, or when you're going to take a break—always pull out slowly. Even if your partner says "Get it out of me now!" don't withdraw too quickly or you can hurt or tear the tender rectal tissue.

As you did with one finger, experiment with different sensations with two fingers. By now your partner should be pretty turned on, so angle your fingers toward the front of the body to hit the G-spot indirectly or the prostate directly. The G-spot and prostate like firm, deliberate stimulation. Use a "come here" motion (almost like a pulling motion) with your fingers to press on the sensitive spot. Because you're putting pressure on the area around the urethra, your partner may feel the urge to pee during G-spot or prostate stimulation. When coupled with arousal, the pee feeling may be pleasurable for some, or annoying for others. Get feedback from your partner about how it feels. In your very first (or first few) anal play experiences, using two fingers is a good goal; two fingers plus other stimulation leading to a rockin' orgasm also works. There will be plenty of time later on for more.

From two fingers, you can progress to three (depending on the size of your fingers) or a slim butt plug or dildo. Remember that you can put a butt plug in, then move on to another activity—vaginal penetration, cunnilingus, mutual masturbation—while the plug works its magic to relax and arouse the ass. When the plug comes out, the ass will be ready for something bigger or longer, or it may be spent. That depends on the ass.

I've outlined a slow, methodical process that may seem like it's a lot of time and effort, which begs the question: Does the receiver always have to warm up for anal penetration? The answer is yes. No matter how experienced you are, you always must begin with fingers or small toys before moving on to a cock or dildo. However, the amount of time it takes your ass to open up and relax will gradually decrease the more you practice.

Check In

Afterward, have a little debriefing session to review how it went and get feedback you can use for next time. Remind each other about goals you set. *Did I go too fast, did I use enough lube? Was there enough in-and-out movement, or do you want more of just that pressure feeling? What did you like about my fingers versus the butt plug? Is there something I can do differently next time? Do you want more genital stimulation while I'm playing with your butt?* Compliments always feel good—criticism does not. Be generous when you communicate with your partner. If you want to tell her or him about something you didn't like, why not start that conversation with something you did like? But make sure you do talk about what didn't work as well as what did work. There are many elements you need to have a pleasurable, pain-free anal sex experience: lots of foreplay and warm-up, plenty of lubrication, and communication and trust between you and your partner. Communication at all phases of an anal sex experience will ultimately help both partners to articulate their needs, and, ideally, help everyone get what he or she wants out of anal sex.

Penetration with Penises, Dildos, and Bigger Toys

When you're ready to move on to a cock, a strap-on dildo, or a bigger toy, the same rules discussed in the previous section apply. In this section, all the tips and techniques can apply to penetration with a penis or a dildo, so when I use the word *cock* I mean any cock, whether rubber or flesh.

Tips for the Giver

After your partner is warmed up and ready for your cock, your erection must be solid to make anal penetration work. While not a problem for cocks of the silicone variety, if you have a flesh cock, make sure it's stiff. Sometimes, a man can have a semihard penis and manage to "stuff" it into a woman's pussy, but that trick won't work on her ass because the anus is such a tight opening. When you're ready, lubricate your cock and relube her ass. Place your cock at her anal opening and hold it with your hand to help you guide it. Now, you have a few options:

Have her move her body toward your cock (forward or backward depending on your positions), while you guide it inside.

Rub your cock against her opening. This external stimulation should relax the anus. As the sphincter muscles contract, the opening appears to "wink" (open, then closed) at you. As it winks open, take the opportunity to slide in.

Press your cock against her opening and gently push against it (she may want to either relax or bear down in order to let you inside).

Penetrate her ass with your finger, withdraw it, and while her anus is open, gently insert your cock. When you first enter her, just put the head of your cock inside, stop, and stay where you are. Let her sphincter muscles and anus get used to the feeling. Keep your movements slow, gentle, and subtle at first. When she's ready, you can venture farther inside. Sometimes, she will actually suck you inside—when we are aroused, our rectums start to contract and we can often pull a cock right in. If she doesn't suck you in, slide into her very slowly or let her come back or down onto the cock so she can control the entry. Now you can start some slow thrusting. Remember when possible to angle toward the front of the body to aim for the G-spot or prostate. She should tell you if she wants you to go deeper or faster or both. Then, it's simply a matter of exploring what feels good for both of you.

STRAP-ON SEX TIPS

Review the tips for selecting the right dildo harness in chapter 8, and make sure your harness fits snugly. As a woman doing the penetration, you should experiment with different positions (see pages 109–118 for a detailed discussion of positions). I know that the first few times I fucked someone in the ass with a strap-on, I had the person in traditional doggie-style position for several reasons. Doggie-style gives you a clear view of the butthole, so you can see exactly what you're doing, and the position allows for a good angle of penetration toward the G-spot or prostate. It's also an easy position in which to get your balance, establish a rhythm, and get some good thrusting going. So, you may want to start out that way, but you can also try any of the other positions in this chapter.

Learning how to skillfully wield a strap-on takes practice and patience. If you feel like the dildo is moving around too much or it doesn't feel secure, then your harness isn't tight enough and you should adjust it. In the beginning, you may want to guide the dildo with your hand, which will give you more control of exactly where it's going. When your partner is ready for penetration, be gentle and go slowly. Press the tip of the well-lubricated dildo against the opening, and have your partner come back on it. This may help him or her feel less vulnerable and more in control of the pace. Once you are inside, and the receiver is ready for some movement, begin slowly. You want to establish a thrusting motion with your hips, one that feels good to your partner and won't tire you out too quickly.

As a woman, you can enjoy penetrating a man or another woman on many different levels. The trust and intimacy between you can feel especially heightened and very arousing. The naughty, taboo aspects of both anal sex and a woman with a dick can really get your motor going. The power she feels as the penetrating partner can also add to your fantasy and pleasure. Plus, strap-on anal sex has the potential to be physically stimulating for you. (Again, see discussion of strap-ons in chapter 8.)

A word to novices: like just about everything else, it takes practice. So, all you guys out there who are thrilled at the idea of a girl with a cock doing

ASK THE ANAL ADVISOR: *Going for the Gape*

Q: My partner really enjoyed something that I unknowingly did last night. I was in doggie-style position, and he was playing with my ass from behind. I was very, very aroused and without knowing or trying, I experienced what I have seen in some porn movies: the gape. It turned him on a great deal. I was able to continue this for quite a while, even while alternating contracting and relaxing my sphincter muscles. Then, suddenly, I just couldn't reproduce the gape again no matter how I tried. If you have any information on how I might cultivate or encourage this skill, I would be most grateful.

A: It sounds to me like you stumbled upon something that other people work pretty hard to achieve! In the adult industry, "the gape" is the postfucking state of openness of an ass. People write to me about seeing the gape in porn videos all the time, but usually it's in fear. They think that once they have anal sex, their ass will end up like a giant pink hole, they'll lose control of their bowel movements, and the anal sphincter muscles will forever stay open. Of course, this isn't the case. I often reassure people that what they are seeing is the ass "at play"—it's just had something quite big pounding away at it, so it's naturally very relaxed, aroused, and ajar. If you saw the same asshole "at rest," it would be small, closed, and puckered as you: have some patience while she practices her technique, remember the first time you used that tool of yours, and give her a break while she figures hers out. And all you women fucking with dildos: make sure you talk to your partner, ask what she or he likes, and try different positions (like those discussed later in this chapter) to see what works best for both of you.

Tips for the Receiver

When your partner is about to enter you, take several deep breaths. Deep breathing will help you relax and concentrate on opening your ass as well as circulating blood to your genitals. (Taking shallow breaths tightens the muscles and inhibits the engorgement process.) Spreading your ass cheeks and holding them apart can help your partner during initial penetration. If you feel yourself start to tense, concentrate on relaxing those sphincter muscles. You may want to relax and bear down slightly.

usual. Your question is an interesting one because you want to achieve the gape, whereas most folks are freaked out by it.

In my experience, some women gape quite easily, others gape only after a prolonged intense ass-fucking, and others rarely if ever get a gape going. Some of it is pure chance; it has to do with how the body responds to penetration, and in particular how the ass behaves after extensive stimulation. Usually in order to get the gape, you need to be very turned on (as you said you were) and have an extended anal penetration scene to get your sphincter muscles to relax and open up. From the description of your experience, you have a good awareness of and control over those muscles, which can also help you go for the gape. In addition to trying to contract and relax the sphincters, you may also want to try to bear down slightly, and see what effect that produces. After your partner pulls out, you can reach around and spread your asscheeks with both hands, which will give the illusion of an open ass. Continuous penetration of some kind may be the key to extending the gape for you, since it sounds like, at some point, the banging stopped, and you were just flexing your muscles. If your partner continues to play with your ass, thus stimulating the area, I bet you'll be able to extend the gape.

It sounds like the opposite of what you should be doing, but it can actually help make penetration easier and more comfortable. Your partner should stimulate your clit or you can self-stimulate as you are penetrated, which will help keep your arousal level up and make penetration more pleasurable.

If your partner is having trouble hitting the intended target (hey, those two holes are close together and it's slippery with all that lube), wrap your fingers around the head of the cock and help guide it inside your ass. Continue to give your partner cues and directions about what you're experiencing and what you need.

Double Penetration

Some women really like the feeling of having both orifices penetrated at the same time. This can be done with fingers, fingers and a toy, two toys, a penis and a toy, or two penises. If you're using a toy, make sure it's made of a flexible material. Some women can accommodate something in their pussy and in their ass simultaneously with relative ease. For others, it takes some effort, lots of warm-up, and practice. It may also depend on the size of the things you're trying to fit in. If you want two penises or two dildos, you may not be able to do it at all, since double penetration really depends on your internal map, and if there's room for two. For most women, when something sizable goes in one hole, the membrane that separates the vaginal and rectal cavities gives slightly one way or the other to accommodate it. So, if there's a large toy in your pussy, your ass may feel tighter than normal (and vice versa).

You can try different techniques to see which one suits you. You may want to inch one finger or cock in one hole, then inch a finger in the

Their penises moved in unison inside me. I could clearly feel them both, their tips meeting, brushing each other through what felt like a flimsy membrane, a thin wall of skin which was in danger at every thrust, and was becoming more and more fragile. They're going to tear me, I thought, they're going to tear me and then they really will meet, one against the other. I repeated it to myself. I liked hearing myself say it. They're going to tear me. What a delicious idea...

—ALMUDENA GRANDES—

other hole. Work your way in slowly, and alternate between the two until it feels comfortable. Or you can have one orifice fully penetrated (the ass would be the best choice since, for most women, it requires more warm-up), then have your partner work his or her way into the other. Some people like to alternate holes—as a finger or a cock goes in one hole, another finger or cock comes out of the other hole—then switch, so the effect is like two pistons going in opposite directions.

You are the one who will know best if it's possible, so make sure you're the one who's in charge and calling the shots. You're testing the limits of your body, so make sure you give your partner plenty of feedback about how it feels.

Anal Sex Positions

People ask me: "What's the best position for anal sex?" My answer: the one that works for both of you. Missionary position can be great, unless keeping her legs in the air or over your shoulders isn't comfortable for her. Spooning works if your bodies line up naturally, and the giver can get a good angle. If you choose doggie-style (my personal favorite), you can do traditional on-all-fours or do head-down, ass-in-the-air. All the positions people employ for vaginal penetration can be used for anal penetration. Since everyone has individual needs, tastes, and desires, it is important to explore all kinds of positions to discover what works best for you and your partner. Think of each new position as an opportunity to explore different depths, speeds, rhythms, and dynamics; there's lots of erotic territory to find simply by changing your point of view.

Missionary Position

This position finds the receptive partner on her or his back and the insertive partner on top; many times, you can enhance this position with a pillow or something like the Liberator Shapes wedge, a firm pillowlike shape designed for sex. Here are a few styles of missionary:

MISSIONARY WITH KNEES UP: Receiver lies on her/his back with giver sitting or kneeling between receiver's legs. To insure full access to the back door, prop up the butt (in order to tip the hips up and back slightly) and have your partner spread her/his legs with knees bent.

LEGS OVER SHOULDERS: Receiver lies on her/his back with heels in the air. Legs can be drawn in so that knees touch the chest or flipped over the shoulders. Giver sits or kneels between receiver's legs. Although this position may create a better angle for entry, it is one that even the most flexible among us may find hard to sustain.

MISSIONARY ON THE EDGE: Receiver lies on her/his back at the edge of the bed (or a massage table, a bondage table, a spanking bench, a comfortable stuffed chair) with giver between receiver's legs, either standing or sitting in a chair of the appropriate height.

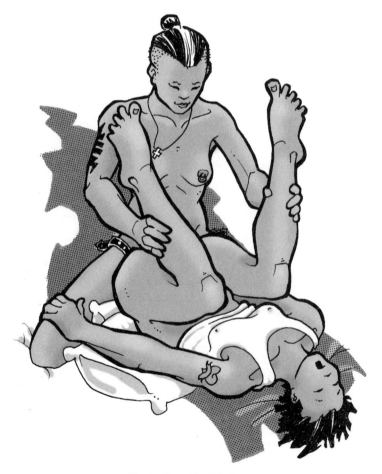

Illustration 12: Missionary

PILE DRIVER: Receiver lies on her/his back, usually on a firm surface like the floor, with nearly entire body below the shoulders pointed upward, and giver standing or squatting for insertion.

Because both partners face each other in these positions, it can be easier to communicate, especially nonverbally, plus you can attend to other parts of your partner's body—suck on her nipples, kiss his neck, nibble her lips. Many people in the receptive position like missionary-style anal penetration because lying on their back either feels more comfortable (except perhaps in the case of Pile Driver) or allows them a sense of surrendering to their partner. In this position, your partner usually cannot provide clitoral or cock stimulation, but you can provide your own with your hand or a vibrator.

Ask the Anal Advisor: *Pain-Free Position*

Q: *My husband and I want to try out anal sex really bad, but my problem is the pain—I know it's not supposed to hurt, but it does. I keep telling him that missionary position is not the best for our first try. Is there another position you recommend? I really want to give this to him, but I am still very nervous.*

A: You admitted being nervous about getting fucked in the ass, which is very common, but my question is: do you really want to do it? I sense some reservation in your letter, and I am concerned that your fear and anxiety may be holding you back. Your desire for this must absolutely be there (not just your husband's), otherwise it's not going to work, and it will continue to hurt. You are right that it is not supposed to hurt, and pain can be the result of many things: hesitation on your part; not being relaxed; not enough foreplay and warm-up; not enough lube. You need to take it slow, and have him open your ass with fingers or small toys before he even attempts to put his cock in there. As for positions, if missionary isn't working for you, trust your instincts. Maybe you should get on top, so you can control the depth of penetration and speed, and you can move your body to get the best angle. Or you could try doggie-style, but make sure he doesn't thrust all the way inside on the first time around.

Receiver on Top

In the receptive-partner-on-top position, the receiver straddles the giver. For example:

ON TOP: Partners face each other, so they can talk and communicate as well as stroke, rub, pinch, and stimulate other parts of each other's bodies; this position allows the giver easy access to the receiver's body for clitoral or cock stimulation.

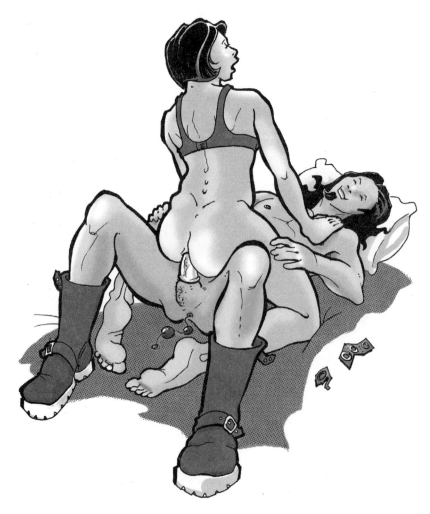

Illustration 13: On Top

REVERSE COWGIRL/COWBOY: This position is identical to On Top, except the partners face the same direction. Depending on the particular curve of the cock or dildo, some receivers prefer this to the original On Top, plus they can stimulate their own genitals. Communication may be tougher in this position, especially if it's your first time.

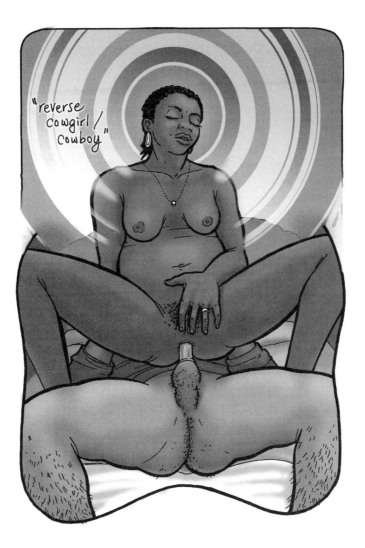

Illustration 14: Reverse Cowgirl/Cowboy

When the receiver is on top, she or he can sit straight up, or lean forward or backward to create the perfect angle. Receptive partners can really take the lead in this position and be in charge of the angle and depth of insertion, the amount of movement, and the rhythm of the penetration. Givers who are inexperienced, nervous about how to penetrate their partners anally, or fearful of hurting their partners may find this position most relaxing because the receiver can do much of the decision making and work. The partner on the bottom often likes this position best because you get a great view of your partner and can watch him or her as he or she receives pleasure.

Doggie-Style (From Behind)

The doggie-style position is probably the first one many of us think of when we think about anal sex. This position, with the receptive partner on her/his hands and knees and the insertive partner behind her/him, has a few variations:

DOGGIE-STYLE ON ALL FOURS: With receiver on hands and knees, giver kneels behind (if on the bed) or stands behind (if using edge of the bed or other furniture).

DOGGIE-STYLE WITH HEAD DOWN: Same as Doggie-Style on All Fours, except receiver's head and shoulders are down. This angles the body perfectly for the giver to hit the G-spot or the prostate.

FLAT FROM BEHIND: The receptive partner is on her or his stomach with knees either bent or straight, the giver lies on top. Although this one may seem awkward on first try, it just takes a little practice. This, too, is a good position for medium or deep penetration because the rectum is in an optimum position for smooth entry.

DOGGIE BENT OVER FURNITURE: Receiver is bent over a bed, couch, or table with giver standing behind.

Doggie-style positions are good for beginner givers, especially if they are trying to navigate between two holes (the vaginal opening and the anal opening). Penetration from behind is best for deep penetration because the rectum is in the most straight (not bent) position, so the insertive partner can get good depth that is also comfortable to the receiver. With doggie-style, you can get a great angle to hit her G-spot or his prostate, as well as reach around to stimulate the clitoris, pussy, or cock. Doing it doggie-style also means both partners can have lots of pelvic movement. The insertive partner can do a lot of deep, hard, or fast thrusting; the receptive partner can move

The ass is a gift. When a woman kneels with her ass in the air, head well down, she feels erotic dread grow in the pit of her stomach and spread through her loins. She can want for this and fear it. In my anticipation of the entry thrust, my heart beats faster, the walls of my vagina swell. It's all up to him. How will he take me?
—SUSAN CRAIN BAKOS—

back on or ride a cock from this angle. Many people like to have their partner penetrate them from behind for a fast and frenzied kind of fuck. As when the receptive partner is on top, she or he can also be in control of the action if the insertive partner does less of the movement and lets the receiver come to him or her.

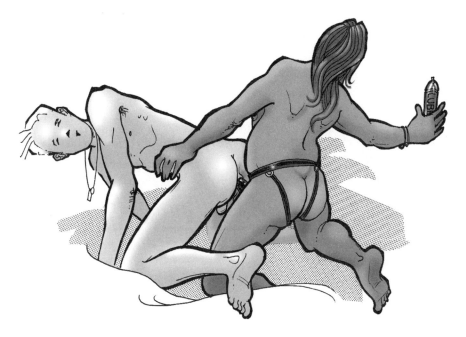

Illustration 15: Doggie-Style

Spooning and Reverse Spooning

In the spooning position, both partners are on their sides either facing each other or facing the same direction. This position is comfortable, flexible, and easily maneuverable, and it gives both partners good control over the angle and depth of penetration; it's an ideal position for partners who are of very different heights or sizes. Some people find that lying side by side gives them greater access to their partner's vagina, clitoris, penis, balls, and more for exploration and stimulation.

You don't get the depth of penetration in spooning that you get with other positions; however, spooning is good for a long, slow anal fucking session, where no one's in a rush to get somewhere. Don't get me wrong—you can still have ecstatic orgasms this way.

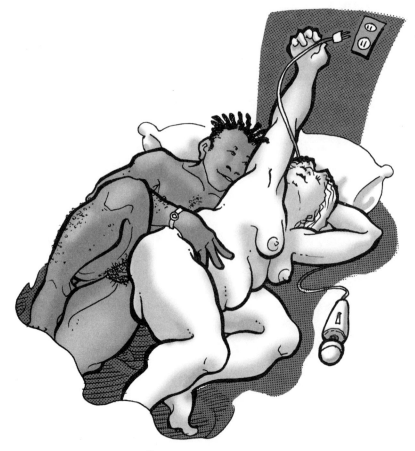

Illustration 16: Spooning

Slings and Swings

Many people find a sling or a swing ideal for anal sex. Slings and swings must be suspended from a weight-bearing beam in the ceiling or a metal stand built specifically to hold it, which can be purchased separately. Lying in one can be both comfortable and extremely supportive, plus your partner can have flexible access to your ass. While you may get into a variety of positions, the key to making this work is having the swing or sling at the proper height so your bodies line up.

ASK THE ANAL ADVISOR: *Can't Get Past the Head*

Q: *My partner likes anal sex very much; she has had plenty of experience and we practice it regularly. But, despite extended warm-up sessions and a lot of lube and communication, she cannot accommodate my penis every time. I am always very gentle and caring. I know that each day with a partner is unique and different even if the mood and environment are the same. The situation is even more frustrating for me (and probably for her too) as we often have to stop after the tip of my cock has gotten inside her. It's almost like some sort of reflex in her body just "rejects" me. What is the best way to achieve full anal sphincter relaxation, allowing an easy and guaranteed penis insertion?*

A: There are no guarantees in life, especially with matters of the heart and ass. It sounds to me like your partner's body isn't relaxed enough, which is why her ass is rejecting you. A surefire solution is to increase the amount of foreplay. I suggest more warm-up with fingers and toys. Add clitoral stimulation to the mix. Using a vibrator, your hand, or hers to manually stimulate her clit while you play with her ass can increase her arousal and help her rectum expand for penetration. Once you first get inside her, don't make any sudden moves. Stay put and give her a chance to adjust to the feeling before you start moving in and out. When she feels relaxed, then start with gentle thrusting, and let her call the shots in terms of speed and depth. Take your time, listen to her body, and don't put so much pressure on yourself and her to make it happen every time.

A sling is like a hammock seat designed especially for sex, and it is usually made of solid, webbed, or crisscrossed leather or nylon. Most come with separate stirrups or ankle and leg cuffs to support your weight, which makes keeping your legs up in the air practically effortless. Some come with a separate piece for head and neck support.

The Love Swing and The Bungee Sexperience Sex Swing are examples of swings. Both basically consist of an adjustable nylon sex harness with straps to support the back and butt or waist and knees, depending on the position you're in. Padded stirrups for feet, ankles, calves, or thighs make it comfortable to be in, even for a long session. You can get into dozens of different positions with a swing, and create different sensations in each. The giver can pull the receiver (the one in the swing) effortlessly back and forth or bounce him or her up or down. The receiver can create the same effect with a slight hip action while his or her partner lies, sits or stands completely still.

Slings and swings are available at specialty sex and leather stores (see Resource Guide).

QUOTES AND SIDEBARS

Rose White and Eric Albert, "She Gets Her Ass Fucked Good" in *Best American Erotica 1997,* edited by Susie Bright (New York: Simon & Schuster, 1997), 82.

Betty Dodson, Ph.D., *Orgasms for Two: The Joy of Partnersex* (New York: Harmony Books, 2002), 189-190.

Almudena Grandes, *The Ages of Lulu,* translated by Sinia Soto (New York: Grove Press, 1994), 184.

Susan Crain Bakos, *Kink,* 10.

CHAPTER 12

Anal Pleasure for Men

While this book says *for women* on the cover, I know that men bought the first edition, as did women who wanted to learn to give pleasure to their male partners. Since our anorectal anatomy is so similar, nearly all the tips and techniques you've read so far throughout the book apply to men as well. You can use your mouth, your fingers, or a sex toy to stimulate or penetrate your man's ass. If you're interested in using a strap-on dildo, follow the recommendations in chapters 8 and 11. In this chapter, I'll cover some of the particular issues—both physical and psychological— that relate specifically to men receiving anal pleasure.

Let me admit my bias about male anal pleasure right off the bat. Getting fucked in the ass is one of the greatest gifts a man can give himself and his partner. First, there is the purely physical prize that awaits him when he is on the receiving end of anal pleasure: those nerve endings, that sensitive tissue, and the unique prostate stimulation. Anal sex is an opportunity for men to be penetrated—a chance to experience pleasure from the other side of the fence, for those usually dishing it out. But in order to access this ecstasy, most men must first get over a lot of shame and fear and embrace all the ass has to offer, which can be easier said than done.

Gender Roles and Psychology

Since anal pleasure is still taboo in American culture, anyone who admits to being a Backdoor Betty is on the front lines of sexual liberation. As women, since we are already positioned as the receptive, penetrated partner, we need only reorient ourselves to focus on the *other* orifice. A man, on the other hand, is seen as the penetrator, the active partner, the pencil to her sharpener. Giving his body over to a woman in a whole new way requires extreme trust, but before he can go there, he's got to deal with some of the baggage that comes with a desire for anal pleasure. Men must confront the stereotype that dudes who like their asses played with are gay. Or the myth that a man has got to be a passive wuss to get fucked in the ass; that real men don't get done up the butt, and if they do, they've somehow put their masculinity in jeopardy. All of this is, of course, bullshit, but that doesn't mean it's easy to let go of and get over.

Over the years, I've received thousands of letters from and spoken face-to-face with hundreds of men who love to get fucked in the ass. Most of them identify as heterosexual and have female partners. Wanting to experience anal pleasure does not make a man gay, kinky, or weird. It doesn't make him less of a man, either. In fact, I think a willingness to embrace a desire that's outside the norm is the sign of a sexually confident, adventurous, open-minded man.

That said, different men like to be fucked in different ways. It's okay if a guy's anal desires involve being submissive, being naughty, or being "forced" (by prior consent) to do it. On the other hand, a guy doesn't have to be passive or submissive to be penetrated. I have personally fucked plenty of men without flipping them—it's all in the way you play it. Encourage your male partner to work through any issues he may have about his sexual or gender role, and to come out of an altogether different closet, along with all the other straight men who can proudly say, "I love getting fucked in the ass!"

Not only can men challenge their gender roles, but so can women. Women who give men anal pleasure can try out the role of active penetrator; we can slip our tongues, fingers, and cocks inside our male lovers'

ANAL PLEASURE FOR MEN • 121

bodies, learning how to give and get pleasure in a brand-new way. Being on the other end of the dick gives women a chance to have their own revolution, too. We can see how the other half does it, and experience our power as women in a new way. This new sexual role alone can be a huge turn-on for some women. There are also plenty of ways for a woman to get physical stimulation while fucking someone with a strap-on (as discussed in chapters 8 and 11).

Prostate Stimulation

Too many men still have not experienced the wonders of their prostate gland. For many of them, their first foray into the land of anal penetration (if they've had one at all) probably took place in a sterile white room, on a paper-covered table. The proctologist squeezed a lump of K-Y onto his latex-clad hand and shoved his finger up your man's ass. It wasn't erotic, it didn't feel particularly good, and your boyfriend wasn't even attracted to the guy. All of this happened five minutes after words like *prostate cancer* and *rectal exam* were uttered. Some turn-on. Now he knows how you feel at the gynecologist. If this is the case for your guy, he needs to put this experience out of his mind—it was a medical exam. I'm talking about mind-blowing sex.

Recall that the prostate sits around a part of the urethra and is about 2 to 3 inches inside the rectum on the front wall. If you slip your finger inside a man's ass and head toward the front of his body, you'll find an area (about the size of a walnut) that feels differently textured than the rest of the rectal wall. At first, you should gently rub the spot as your partner gives you feedback about how it feels. Every guy is different, so your partner's communication is critical to helping you stimulate him in exactly the way he wants. As he gets more aroused, the prostate will swell and become more sensitive. It can also handle more firm and deliberate stimulation once it's swollen, and you can employ some of the same techniques I've described for stimulating the G-spot throughout the book. For prostate stimulation with a dildo (whether strapped on or in your hand), select a curved toy and make sure the curve is always toward the front of his body.

Some guys like to have their cocks and balls played with, while others want anal play alone—that's something for the two of you to experiment

He clamps up to prevent me from
rubbing here, but aggression has
risen in me and I press on, massaging
a moistened finger at the entrance.
It's slick there, and I can imagine the
smell, which excites me; I know that
he's concerned about the smell, too—
how I'll find him—and this excites
me. The thought pops into my mind
that if I had a dick, right now if I had
a dick, I would wear him out..."
—MAGENTA MICHAELS—

with. When some men have their ass stimulated, they may lose their erection. There are several theories about why this can happen. As a man relaxes his pelvic and sphincter muscles to allow penetration, the pelvic region is too relaxed to maintain an erection. Some men get entirely focused on the stimulation of their ass, and their cock is not the focal point of the pleasure. Don't be alarmed if it happens to your partner. A loss of erection could signal a man's fear or anxiety about being penetrated, and you may want to check in with your partner if you sense some physical or emotional discomfort. However, a man may also be having the time of his life and still have a less than rock-hard cock. It may not happen every time he is penetrated, or it may change as he becomes aroused. Worrying about his loss of erection is not going to help it return or help either of you to have a good time. Relax, and let it do whatever it wants to do.

Just for Men: The Aneros

The Aneros is a unique anal toy that looks like a butt plug with two thin, curled handles on the base; there are five different styles of the Aneros that vary slightly in size or design (see illustration 10 in chapter 8). The Aneros was designed specifically for prostate massage and is prescribed as a medical treatment for men with prostate problems. It's also a really cool sex toy you can encourage your male partner to use alone or with you. After warmup with a finger or two, insert the well-lubed Aneros into the ass, making sure that the loop of the base that curves up (referred to in the instructions as the "perineum abutment") is positioned to press against the perineum (the area between the anus and the scrotum). Once he's used to having it inside him, tell him to begin contracting his sphincter muscles. Don't use your hand to move the toy, tell him to use only his muscles. These contractions

Ask the Anal Advisor: *Convince My Wife, Please*

Q: *I love it when my wife wears a strap-on and gives it to me in the butt. My problem is that she only does it occasionally. I wish she would do it more and enjoy it more. Any suggestions?*

A: Since you've already gotten your ass plowed by her before, I think it's fair to ask her directly why you're not getting the backdoor gift from her more often. Have you asked her directly why she might be hesitant to do it? Have you told her how much it turns you on? Your wife may have some issues with being the penetrator (instead of the penetrated), since it is not a straight woman's typical role; however, you can reassure her that there are plenty of other women giving it to their guys and loving every minute of it. Many people can buy into the myth that if men want to be fucked in the ass, then they are really gay. This is ridiculous, of course. In most cases, men who identify as heterosexual and enjoy giving and/or receiving anal sex with women are not repressing gay desires. Your wife may be a victim of this stereotype, and you need to assure her that you love her, are attracted to her, and want her alone to do you in the ass. Perhaps she hasn't realized her own potential for pleasure during strap-on sex. In addition to being a real turn-on upstairs (in her head), having her cock in your ass provides plenty of ways for her to get off.

actually move the toy inside him, pushing the head of it into the prostate and creating pleasurable stimulation of the nerve endings. Simultaneously, the abutment presses on the perineum, stimulating it as well. Aneros toys are nonporous, and makers recommend using water-based lube with them; they can be cleaned with hot water and antibacterial soap.

A Different Kind of Orgasm

Men can definitely have orgasms as a result of anal penetration. Some men add cock stimulation (you can stimulate his penis or he can do it himself) to anal penetration, and can come from the combination. Others can come from just a good ass-fucking. Other men may experience a different kind of orgasm from prostate stimulation than they do from having their penis stimulated manually, orally, or via penetration. Many men report that they have a prostate orgasm—all the sensations of an orgasm without ejaculation. Or they may climax and ejaculate a clear fluid that's different looking than their usual ejaculate—this is prostatic fluid, the fluid produced by the prostate gland. So, there are many possibilities, and it may be a matter of both of you reorienting around a different expectation of an orgasm.

QUOTE

Magenta Michaels, "Taking Him on a Sunday Afternoon" in *Herotica 2: A Collection of Women's Erotic Fiction,* edited by Susie Bright and Joani Blank (San Francisco: Down There Press, 1991), 19.

CHAPTER 13

BDSM and Anal Play

BDSM: The Basics

BDSM is an abbreviation of sorts that represents three distinct but related terms: B & D (bondage and discipline), D/s (Dominance and submission), and S/M (sadism and masochism or sadomasochism). BDSM is meant to be a catchall term that encompasses all the activities for which the letters stand and more. Erotic but not necessarily sexual, BDSM is an intimate experience, an exchange of power between people that may be physical, psychological, spiritual, or all of the above. Common BDSM activities include bondage, flogging, spanking, sensory deprivation, sensation play, and Dominant/submissive role-play. If you've ever played with handcuffs or blindfolds, controlled or punished someone, or explored the line between pleasure and pain during sex, then you've done BDSM.

In BDSM, the top is the person who is in charge, initiates action, and does things to the bottom; the bottom follows the top's lead, receives action, and has things done to him or her. In general, but not always, tops like to control and run the show, and bottoms like to give up control and surrender. Simply put, tops do, bottoms get done. Many tops are dominant—their needs and wishes come first, and many bottoms are submissive—their desire is to please and serve the Dominant. However, that is not always the case. For example, if a dominant Master orders his submissive to flog him, then the Master is the flogging bottom and the submissive is the flogging top; the Master is still the one in charge, he's just having something done to him. People may also identify with multiple roles, including both top and bottom, and they are called switches.

Because BDSM encompasses so many different practices, kinky people like to talk with their partners first about their likes and dislikes. Negotiation is one of the basic tenets of BDSM and one that everyone (no matter if you're kinky or not) can learn from. Good negotiation requires you to determine what you want, be able to communicate it, and then make it happen. Once each partner lays down the ground rules for what they want and don't want, what's okay and what's not, both need to respect each other's physical and emotional boundaries.

Negotiation prior to any BDSM scene is crucial. It's especially important for the top (the doer) to have as much information as possible about the experience level of the bottom (the one who gets done). The idea is to have as much knowledge as you can before the scene, so you can plan

---

BDSM Terminology

PLAY: equivalent to practicing BDSM, as in "I played with him last week."

SCENE: when two (or more) people come together to do BDSM.

TOP: one who dishes it out.

BOTTOM: one who takes it.

SWITCH: one who likes to dish it out and take it, depending on the circumstances.

SADIST: one who derives pleasure from inflicting physical and/or emotional pain and discomfort on others.

MASOCHIST: one who enjoys receiving that pain and/or discomfort.

accordingly. Here are some examples of questions about anal play that a top might ask a bottom:

How much experience have you had with BDSM?

How much experience have you had with anal play?

Are you sensitive or allergic to latex or any kinds of lube?

When was the last time you did any kind of anal play and what was it?

What are your turn-ons and turn-offs when it comes to your ass?

How much warm-up does your ass need and what works best for you?

What's the biggest thing you've ever had in your ass (and when did it happen)?

The bottom should be as specific as possible in all his or her answers. For example, if the response to the question "What's the biggest thing you've ever had in your ass?" is "Something really big," ask the person to be more specific: big like a cucumber or big like a watermelon? Knowing this type of information will help you figure out about how long the scene will last, decide what toys to bring, and determine what kinds of warm-up you'll do.

You should both agree to use a safeword during a scene. A safeword is a word—usually one that you wouldn't normally utter during a scene—that you and your partner choose. Since *stop* or *no* or *please don't* may be part of the dialogue of a scene, none of these words or phrases should be your safeword. Your safeword is your safety net. If you don't like something that's happening or you want the scene to stop right away, simply say your safeword.

Lots of different BDSM activities can be combined with anal play, including bondage, sensory deprivation, hot wax, flogging, and piercing.[1] In this chapter, I will discuss specific activities where the ass is a central part of the play, including spanking, butt plug play, anal training, psychological play, Dominance and submission, penetration by consensual force, and erotic enema play.

Spanking

There's nothing like a good old-fashioned spanking. Whether you use your hand, a paddle, or another tool, a series of smacks on someone's ass-flesh can be highly erotic and enjoyable. For some, a spanking is a sensual turn-on. For others, in an erotic context, something that could be painful transforms into pleasure. When the body experiences an intense or painful sensation, it releases endorphins and other chemicals that attempt to inhibit the pain; these hormones may cause you to feel aroused, euphoric, or high. Add a psychological component to the spanking—like imagining yourself or your partner as a naughty boy receiving punishment at the hands of the governess—and you've got an erotic and emotionally-charged scenario.

For novice bottoms and tops and those looking for a light to moderate sensation, it's best to begin with your own hand. Your hand can help gauge just how soft or hard you are hitting someone, and is the easiest of tools to master since you've been using it your entire life. Take off rings and bracelets, which can distract and cause injury, before you spank anyone.

Get your bottom in a comfortable position—for example, lying over your lap, on all fours, or bent over the bed or a table. If you haven't yet done any foreplay or other touching, before you start spanking, it's a good idea to get the bottom going. The more aroused he or she is, the more enjoyable the spanking will be for both of you. So, lick her pussy a little, stroke his cock, talk dirty to her, suck on his nipples, do whatever it is you know will get your bottom nice and turned on.

Talk to your bottom, tell him or her what you're about to do. Perhaps say why you're giving the spanking if it's part of the scene: "You've been a very bad girl," or "This is because you forgot to thank me for untying you." Have the bottom count each smack to help focus on the spanking and anticipate the next lick to come. You can also have the person repeat a phrase like, "Please Mistress, may I have another?" If she or he forgets to say it or miscounts, you can start back at one. Verbal communication will not only keep you connected to one another and the scene, but as the top, you'll be able to determine when you're nearing your bottom's limit by her breathing and the tone in her voice, as well as her body language.

Begin by stroking and kneading the buttcheeks. Rubbing them will help to warm the skin and prepare it for the spanking; plus it will turn your partner on and tempt him or her with what's to come. Slightly cup your hand with the fingers together. Start out very lightly, just tapping the fullest part of the ass; make sure you avoid hitting the tailbone. After this very light spank, gently massage the area you just hit. Begin alternating sides with a light spank, followed by a massage. Keep your hand as close to the ass as possible; the farther away you bring your hand, the less control you have over hitting the exact spot you are aiming for and the more likely you are to hit too hard. You may want to spank with one hand and use the other one to play with her clit or his cock. Genital stimulation will help relax the bottom and make the spanking feel more sensual. Keep it relatively light in the beginning, and don't spank your bottom more than one- or two-dozen times. You can always have a heavier, longer spanking later. If you're going to spank someone and then do something else to his or her ass (flog it, cane it, or drip hot wax on it, for example), keep in mind that after a spanking, the skin is much more sensitive.

When you're ready to try different spanking tools, check your own home for useful things like a wooden spoon, spatula, or hairbrush. Or you may want to invest in a toy called a slapper (two pieces of leather sewn together at one end) or a leather paddle. There are also paddles made of rubber or wood, which deliver a much stronger, harder smack than their leather counterparts. Because slappers and paddles can be made of a variety of materials, it is important to know your tools before you start wielding them on another person. Most of them can produce a light sensation or a heavy, painful one depending on how much force is behind it. There are a variety of brushes made for grooming horses (found at tack stores), which can be used on the ass to create unique tactile feelings. Rub or "brush" the cheeks with them, or, for a heavier feeling, you can actually spank with some of them. The important things is to be very familiar with the implement and what different kinds of sensations it is capable of delivering as well as the pain it may inflict. Test out your spanking tools on your inner thigh before using them on someone else.

A really good spanking begins long before skin-on-skin contact is even made. Often, the atmosphere and context can be even more arousing than the spanking itself, and the prelude to a spanking can be one of the most panty-wetting, cock-stiffening moments of tension you'll ever experience.
—VIOLET BLUE—

Some paddles are leather on one side and soft fur (real or fake) on the other, so you can alternate between a whack and a gentle caress. If you don't have a two-sided paddle, you can use a fur mitt, a fuzzy glove, or a feather to create a similar gentle sensation. Try spanking with one bare hand and one hand wearing a leather glove. To create a combination of hot and cold, rub an ice cube over the ass, making sure to let some water drip between the cheeks. When the asscheeks are wet, the spanking will sting more.

Spanking complements anal play in a scene well, since the attention paid to the bottom's ass—in the form of taps, smacks, slaps, tickles, and other sensations—not only feels good, but helps draw blood to the area, helping the anal arousal process. It's a win-win situation!

Butt Plugs and BDSM

In chapter 8, I extolled the virtues of the butt plug as a sex toy, but it can also be used as a BDSM tool. For the tops: learn to think of a butt plug as your "proxy top," and use it to begin a scene in your absence. Send an email, or leave a voicemail message or a note with the following instructions: *Put the [description here] butt plug in at 5:00 p.m. Whenever you shift or move and feel that plug in your ass, think of [fill in important thing here]. See you at 6:00.* Once the bottom gets this missive, the scene has begun, and you're not even there! I like to give the butt plug a very specific meaning; that way, it accomplishes two tasks simultaneously: it helps the bottom become more aware of his or her ass and forces him or her to think about what's coming later. "Whenever you shift or move and feel that plug in your ass, think of..." The end of this sentence could be any number of things: my cock, the cane, my fist, your hands and legs bound—whatever it is you want the person to begin to anticipate. The possibilities are endless.

After the plug goes in, whether the bottom is at home or running an errand, he or she should be squirming in no time. Having several minutes or hours to ponder one's fate puts a bottom in a good frame of mind; having a plug in your bottom's ass means you don't have to begin at square one—it's already been warming up without you. I received a letter from a submissive whose Mistress wanted him to a wear a bigger plug because it would make him more submissive to her. I told him that a bigger plug would make him more aware of his ass, and, by extension, could help him focus on his dedication and service to his Mistress. But the size of a butt plug alone does not affect one's level of submission, and bigger does not always inspire better. If you would like your partner to wear it for longer than fifteen minutes, review the tips and techniques in chapter 14 for long-term butt plug wear.

Ask the Anal Advisor: *Figging*

Q: *Have you heard of figging? Do you think it's safe to do?*

A: Rumored to have been practiced as early as the Victorian era (they were so kinky!), figging involves sticking a ginger root up someone's (or your own) ass, and most people I know do it in the context of a BDSM scene. The idea is that the ginger elicits an intense, long-lasting, burning sensation in the sensitive, delicate tissue of the rectum. I've heard of some Dominants who insert the root into a submissive's ass before a spanking, paddling, or caning. The longer the root is inside the butt, and the more blood that rushes to the area, the stronger the burning. Plus, any kind of movement—including clenching the sphincter muscles—increases the fiery feeling. This is not an activity for anal play novices or people with extra-sensitive behinds. While some bottoms say that figging feels warm and tingly, most report that the sensation is ten times more intense.

There are a few safety tips that go along with this practice. You should begin with a fresh, whole ginger piece (also called a *hand*), and peel off the brown rough skin before slicing a *finger* to use for penetration. Because it obviously does not have a flared base (and therefore could get lost in the ass), select the largest piece you can find, and either carve out your own shape with a base or attach a string to it in order to make it easy to retrieve. After handling a peeled root, you shouldn't touch your eyes or your partner's eyes. Some figging fans say that lube can seal in the moisture and prevent it from releasing, thereby defeating the purpose, but you know my stance on lube: you need it! Other than those precautions, as with all perverted activities, use your common sense.

Anal Training

Like the use of butt plugs, anal training is a great way to both mentally reinforce the Dominant/submissive dynamic and physically prepare the ass for extended anal play. Anal training can be effective for bottoms who are beginners to anal pleasure or those who want to work their way up to extended play sessions, big toys, or fisting. Slow, methodical anal play, where you progress to the next step only when you've fully enjoyed the

previous step, is a very effective tool. As you have more and more pleasurable experiences, you increase your chances of being able to take more
in your ass for longer. Training can be a top's method of discipline and control over the bottom's body. If a bottom is especially scared, hesitant, or
nervous about anal play, adding a Dominant/submissive training dynamic
to your play can do wonders. A sense of obligation—the bottom needs to
do it for you—can help motivate the bottom to get over his or her fear.
Training brings structure to the experience, where each step is paced, and
the bottom doesn't feel like he or she has to accomplish everything all at
once. When you're able to set attainable goals for the bottom, and he or
she meets those goals, the sense of accomplishment brings with it a
newfound confidence.

If your bottom is nervous about anal play or lives far away from you,
or if you like to give homework assignments, solo anal exercises can be a
useful tool. Nervous bottoms often make more progress on their own at
first because the pressure to please the top is taken out of the mix and they
can focus on themselves. If top and bottom don't see each other often, it
can be difficult to maintain sexual momentum and pick up where you left
off; having the bottom do self-stimulation can keep his or her butt in shape
until the next time you see each other. Assign anal masturbation exercises,
where the bottom must play with fingers, plugs, or dildos on a regular
schedule, track his or her progress, and report back to you.

The training method that I think works best is to set up a plan for the
bottom. Decide if the action is going to be solo or in your presence, then
create a regimen that calls for gradual increases in a number of elements.
First, have the bottom start with one finger, a very small plug, or a slim
dildo and play with it (in the case of the plug, wear it) for fifteen minutes.
If using a toy, it should be something soft and flexible made of either latex,
vinyl, or silicone. Continue the same "small" activity each day, adding fifteen
minutes to the ritual. After a week, switch to two fingers or a toy that's
slightly bigger, and start back at the fifteen-minute mark. Have the bottom
work up to more time for another week. With each week, increase the
size of the toy and the duration of the play session. Anal bead toys and
others that have sections that graduate in size are great tools for training
and tracking progress. Once the bottom reaches your goal, with each new
week after that, instead of changing the size of the plug or dildo, just up
the amount of time. Make sure you allow genital stimulation in addition

to anal play to make the experience more pleasurable. Instruct the bottom that if anything hurts, he or she should go back down to the smaller-size plug, staying with it until he or she feels ready for more.

All the rules of anal play still apply: relaxation, plenty of lube, patience, et cetera. Proper anal training works on several fronts. It can condition the bottom's ass by getting it relaxed, open, and ready for more; plus, it can psychologically condition the bottom to be obedient, focused, and disciplined.

Psychological Play

Psychological play in BDSM is focused on the mind (some people call it mindfuck) and may or may not be combined with other types of play. Tops use mental tools like fear and terror, embarrassment, phobias, verbal abuse, interrogation, humiliation, and objectification to provoke, confuse, shock, intimidate, and elicit various emotions from bottoms. A top may attempt to push emotional buttons, screw with someone's sense of reality, trick, deceive, challenge, or dare a bottom.

In addition to being a physically exciting or intense experience, anal play can be very emotionally and psychologically charged; therefore, it is an ideal activity to incorporate into scenes with a psychological angle. Below I will show how some of the basic characteristics of anal sex I've discussed throughout the book can be used as a starting point to create or enhance a psychological play scene.

Quality: Anal sex is a special, unique activity.
Scene: Ownership, control

For many people, anal sex may be something that they don't do every time they have sex. It may be something they've only done with one person. Taking this attribute to the next level, as a top, you can demand ownership of your bottom's ass. Tell the bottom that she or he cannot touch her or his ass without your permission and no one else can touch it either. The ass becomes a physical symbol of your dominance. You take control of that part of the bottom's body and you become the sole source of the bottom's anal pleasure. You can deny that pleasure for an hour, a day, a week, or a month, or indulge the pleasure as a reward for good behavior.

Quality: Anal sex requires a great deal of trust between partners.
Scene: Dominance and submission, power exchange

There is an inherent power dynamic in the act of penetration. As the penetrator, you are putting part of your body (or some extension of you) into someone else's body. As the penetrated, you're opening up a delicate part of your body and taking something inside you. I believe there is power in both of these roles. The act of anal penetration can be a metaphor for dominance and submission. Fucking someone in the ass could be the ultimate act of dominance; you are invested with the power to enter, invade, and occupy a precious place. You have the power to harm or please. On the flipside, being fucked in the ass can be the ultimate act of submission. You relinquish a delicate, vulnerable part of your body to another person, you lie open and exposed, you surrender to a top's desire, control, and wishes.

Quality: Anal sex can test the boundaries of mind and body.
Scene: Endurance, limit-testing

BDSM can be an exploration of the limits of the body and mind, and anal penetration can be an excellent manifestation of this metaphor. How much can you give? How much can you take? How long can you last? In some cases, the more you take, the more you *want* to be able to take, because once you transcend the fear of having something inside your ass, the sky's the limit.

In my workshops (and in the early chapters of this book), I counter the myths and misinformation that may prevent some people from beginning to explore anal eroticism. Over the years, I've worked with many people to overcome their fears and anxieties about their asses, so they can embrace this special spot as a source of sexual pleasure. This has meant getting over some of the negative baggage that is associated with all things anal. However, for kinky people, we can exploit these very same elements in developing hot mindfucking scenes. As a bottom, these elements aren't just a turn-on, but a way to explore your own boundaries with your top. Anal sex—the promise or the threat of it—can be a wonderful psychological tool. Let's revisit some of the myths from chapter 1 and see how they can be used to our advantage in consensual fantasy scenes.

Myth: Anal sex is dirty and messy.
Scene: Shame, embarrassment, humiliation

In reality, we know that anal sex does not have to be messy at all. However, if your bottom is someone who is fastidiously clean, then you can play with the idea that his or her ass is filthy and disgusting. Use verbal taunts to push his buttons: tease her about soiling your white sheets and having to clean it up. When playing with a neat freak who also enjoys being embarrassed in an erotic context, this can be a great way for a top to make the most of his or her bottom's fear and shame around being dirty.

Myth: Anal sex hurts.
Scene: Fright, danger, infliction of pain

The ass is a delicate area of the body that requires careful handling; in other words, you could hurt someone if you don't do it correctly. Does your bottom like to be scared with the possibility of pain or bodily harm? Does she get turned on by the thought of something dangerous being done to her? Fear is one of our most potent emotions, and one that can also arouse us in the right context. Threatening someone with using no lube, putting huge things in his or her ass without warm-up, or tearing up his or her insides can be part of scenes of terror, intimidation, or interrogation.

Myth: Anal sex is naughty.
Scene: Naughtiness, punishment, discipline

I know a woman who merely needs to hear the words *anal sex,* and she is sent into a blushing state of mortification and arousal. The idea alone makes her feel like she's misbehaving and perverted. If your bottom likes to be a naughty boy or girl, anal sex can feed into a role-playing scene full of teasing, punishment, and other delicious possibilities.

Only a short while before, when she had been kneeling half-naked before René, and Sir Stephen had opened her thighs with both his hands, René had explained to Sir Stephen why O's buttocks were so easily accessible, and why he was so pleased that they had been so prepared: it was because it had occurred to him that Sir Stephen would enjoy having his preferred path constantly at his disposal.

—PAULINE RÉAGE—

Maintaining the D/s Dynamic

In all situations, I recommend lots of communication during anal play, so partners can check in with one another about their needs and wants. But the typical kind of back-and-forth dialogue will not work while you're in Dominant/submissive role-play. A Daddy who's a strict disciplinarian doesn't

ASK THE ANAL ADVISOR: *From a Dominatrix*

Q: *I'm a professional Dominatrix, and I have several clients who've asked me to put strange things in their asses. One who's into forced feminization and anal play requested that I insert tampons into his "pussy" (which is what he likes to call his ass when we play). I know that there is a risk of Toxic Shock Syndrome when tampons are used vaginally, and I am wondering if it can happen in the ass as well. Another brought in this enormous dildo that I just know is never going to go in his ass. What's a Domme to do?*

A: Toxic Shock Syndrome is a blood-borne bacterial infection caused by the bacteria staphylococcus. We most commonly hear about it in relation to using tampons, and symptoms can include fever, chills, vomiting, sore throat, headache, and more serious conditions. It is treated with intra-venous antibiotics to prevent shock and kidney failure. TSS colonizes skin and mucous membranes, and the rectum is a mucous membrane; how-ever, I had a difficult time locating any documented cases of TSS through the use of tampons anally. Since tampons are used to absorb moisture, it could be uncomfortable and dehydrating at the very least. As for the huge dildo client, well, it sounds like he has a syndrome that befalls lots of bot-toms: their eyes are bigger than their orifices. I have an easy solution for you and anyone whose partner wants something in his or her ass that you know is either unsafe or potentially dangerous (like glass bottles, candles, baseball bats, just to name a few). Find a sex toy with a similar size and feel to the desired (but unadvisable) object. Wave the desired toy around, refer to it, talk about it. Then, blindfold your bottom, and do the ol' bait and switch, inserting the similar but far safer toy in the ass. Keep talking about the original object and spin the fantasy. If you're a good Dominant, you can convince a submissive of almost anything.

ask, "How does that feel honey, am I hurting you?" And "Do you want me to put the bigger butt plug in now?" won't work coming from a controlling Mistress. Similarly, a submissive submitting to a Dominant can't direct, "Go slower, I don't like it so fast" or offer "Okay, I'm ready for more now." That kind of banter could throw off the power dynamic both of you want to create and maintain.

So, in addition to prior communication and negotiation, I recommend that tops find creative ways for both partners to communicate during a scene. For example, tell your bottom that when she's ready for another finger, a bigger toy, or whatever the next step is, she needs to *ask* for it, as in: "Sir, may I please have another finger?" You can also insist that she move onto whatever is penetrating her (a dildo, a plug, a penis) so that you've told her what to do, but she can do it at her own pace. Or maybe you're not that nice; in that case, make your bottom *beg* for each new thing. These simple shifts in language or in how you recast the exact same actions in different ways, lets the bottom communicate to the top about what she needs while simultaneously reinforcing the Dominant/submissive dynamic.

Penetration by Consensual Force

It may be rough sex, having penetration forced on the bottom, or acting out a rape fantasy. Whatever the scenario, I use the term "consensual force" deliberately. Force by definition means a lack of consent, but in a fantasy scene, both partners communicate and negotiate terms and limits before the scene, and the bottom consents to the force. Part of why and how consensual force can work is the deep trust between partners and the limits each one sets. The force is on the bottom's terms and either partner knows he or she can stop the scene for any reason. Because of the total submission and surrender to another that anal sex can imply, it can be a very hot part of a consensual force scene.

In one of my favorite scenes, a top put me in elaborate bondage that was a combination of leather restraints, rope, and Ace bandages. I was semimummified in the bandages, and I felt completely confined and nearly immobile. She had me facedown on the bed, and the only part of me exposed was my ass. She threatened to take me; to fuck my ass without warm-up, without lube, and without self-control. She went on and on about how I was going to take her big dick in my ass whether I liked it or not. Luckily for me, she put a butt plug in my ass while she barked at me, which helped me warm up and prepare my ass for its violation. When she took the plug out, I was ready for that big dick. As she was fucking me, she continually scolded me for being so naughty and wanting to be tied up

Ask the Anal Advisor: *Pain on Purpose*

Q: *Receiving anal penetration and being sexually submissive have always been the focus of my sexual fantasies. More specifically, I like the anal penetration to be painful. We usually start with fingers, dildos, or plugs, but unlike everything else I've read, we use these to make me sore, not to warm me up, and we use as little lubrication as possible. I can only feel totally aroused when it begins to burn, sting, or ache and I feel I want my partner to stop. This particular pain, coupled with some light to medium flogging, is the one thing that makes me really orgasm. I also love the feeling of soreness the next day. I always recover after a day or so of restraint, but I am now worried after reading more about the do's and don'ts of anal sex that over time I could cause permanent damage to myself.*

A: It's incredibly brave of you to be so honest about your sexual desires and practices, especially when many people might see them as wrong and politically incorrect, even fellow BDSM players. I appreciate your candor, and I think that yours is an important letter, because I am sure you are not the only one out there. As kinky people who practice all kinds of BDSM, we know that there is a fine line between pleasure and pain, and that line is different for everyone. People who enjoy flogging, spanking, piercing, and other forms of intense sensation play know the high we get from the rush of endorphins, the thrill of pushing the limits of our bodies, and the orgasmic potential of these activities which nonkinky people may see as cruel and painful. As a community, BDSM players often reiterate ad nauseam that our activities are "safe, sane, and consensual" and we frown upon unsafe players. With most forms of sensation play, you can paddle, whip, beat, pierce, and cut fleshy, well-padded areas of the body. You should never strike joints, boney areas, areas around internal organs, the neck, head, or face.

and fucked in the ass. She was rough and nasty, and the frenetic energy of the scene was really hot. The best part was that I could surrender to anal sex "against my will," but still have the trust and safety because I knew my top would take care of me.

I think the anus would fall into the latter category as an area we shouldn't deliberately hurt. Unlike fleshy parts of our body that may redden, bruise, or bleed but eventually recover completely, the ass is not so resilient. The rectum is quite delicate, which is why sex educators like myself encourage people to go slow, warm the body up, and use plenty of lube. It's a matter of comfort—I assume that the majority of people do not want to experience pain through anal penetration. Anal sex has long been mythologized as violent and painful for women, and I am attempting to counteract that stereotype by teaching people to have pain-free anal penetration.

Your desire for pain puts you in the minority, but that doesn't mean it is not valid. However, you need to know the risks of your practices. Through repeated penetration with little warm-up, no lube, or deliberate roughness, you can scrape or abrade the rectum, develop anal fissures, put yourself at risk for STD transmission, and cause permanent damage to your ass. Permanent damage could mean no more anal play at all, which doesn't sound like what you want. Yours is a difficult dilemma. I want you to do what turns you on and makes you come, but I don't want you to hurt yourself or damage your body in the process. I think you should explore other kinds of play that produce similar sensations for you, but happen on a less fragile part of the body. But even as I write that recommendation, I realize that part of the turn-on for you may be that you don't want to feel pain in the "safe" places on your body, but rather in the very places we're told are too delicate and off limits. You and your partner should explore new ways to approximate the pain sensations while still taking good care of your ass. For example, adding warm-up and lube to the equation will protect your body and won't necessarily prevent you from feeling the burn or the ache, especially with larger toys. You need to find that unique line for yourself where the sensation is intense enough to satisfy you, but you are mindful of not hurting yourself.

Scenes with mutually agreed upon forced sex of any kind, and especially those with forced anal sex, are delicate, complex, and tricky; they require a tremendous amount of trust between partners and plenty of prior negotiation. Before the scene begins, you and your partner should talk about what is okay and what isn't. Tops: reassure your bottom that she is free to use her safeword at any time if things aren't going well for her. As a top, remember that the goal is to use dominance and control with physical and psychological elements to create the fantasy for the bottom. Be sure your bottom is specific about the vibe of the scene. Does she want to feel a sense of surrender, of being taken against her will? Does she want to feel used, degraded, or humiliated? Does she want to be verbally abused? Ask if there are any particular words, actions, or scenarios that may trigger someone in a negative way; for example, I know a woman who suffered physical abuse as a child. As an adult, she likes to be spanked with a variety of implements *except* wooden spoons. For some people, yelling cannot be part of a rough scene. The idea is for both people to approach each other with respect and responsibility. Realize that setting these limits and discussing them beforehand still may not prevent someone from having an emotional response during a scene: be prepared so that if something comes up, you will be there to support your partner.

In addition to prior negotiation, creative communication during the scene also plays a big role, since the victim can't say "slow down" or "that hurts" when she is supposed to be at the mercy of her captor; likewise, the captor can't say "how are you doing?" or "is this okay?" as he tortures his victim.

As the top, you can threaten to have your way with her, fuck her without lube, and rip her a new asshole, but in reality, no anal penetration should happen without working your way up. BDSM can be a way to explore the edges of pleasure and pain, but these practices should never be confused with anal sex being painful. Anal sex shouldn't hurt at all; if it does, you're not using enough lube or you're rushing it. Actually forcing anal penetration can cause damage to the delicate lining of the anus and rectum. But in this kind of scene, you don't necessarily want to begin with a gentle finger and your usual foreplay routine. One solution I recommend: have the bottom do her own warm up, which may include wearing a butt plug for some length of time, before the scene. This way, her ass is prepared for some heavy play when she arrives. (For tips on long-term butt plug wear, see chapter 14.)

That still doesn't mean that you can stick your giant cock inside her right off the bat, however. You'll have to figure out imaginative ways to warm up her ass even as you're forcing yourself on her. Here's where I employ a technique I call "I'm going to stick every single thing in this room up your ass." I carefully place two kinds of items around the room: ones I will use (small, medium, large toys) and ones I will only threaten to use (wine bottles, plungers, nightsticks). As the scene progresses, I give the illusion that I am grabbing anything in sight and sticking it into my bottom's butt; in reality, I have carefully planned the order of each toy. I create the sense of urgency, of sexual use, of taking her, while still taking care of my bottom in a responsible way. The trick is to capture the spirit of force, degradation, and surrender, while still maintaining the principles of safety: be patient, go slow, use lots of lube, and listen to the bottom's verbal and nonverbal cues.

With any highly-charged scene like this one, be prepared for emotions to be intense and issues to come up. No matter how much you prepare and communicate beforehand, either partner can experience intense feelings like rage, sadness, and fear during a scene like this. Be prepared to stop if you need to, and make time to check in with one another afterward.

Erotic Enema Play

For some, an enema is a means to an end, a cleansing ritual and that's all. For others, it's a very erotic experience, and there are plenty of websites, erotic stories, and videos devoted to erotic enema play that prove that the desire is not uncommon. Some people get off on the sensation an enema creates. Think about it: water rushing into your ass is another form of penetration, and there are plenty of butt plug–like nozzles to enhance the penetration. An erotic enema can be part of fantasy role-playing, like a medical scene with a nurse and patient or an "age play" scene where one partner plays a kid and the other an authoritative figure like Daddy, Mommy, or a nanny. These scenes often involve some form of regression back to a helpless, innocent, or primal state where the bathroom is the site of shame, curiosity, and growth and toilet training is a highly-charged ritual. Giving someone an enema can be part of different BDSM scenes to symbolize a Dominant's control over his or her submissive's body and bodily functions, to reinforce someone's submission, to humiliate or shame someone, or to inflict intentional discomfort. If you're going to engage in the latter—give someone a cold water enema to produce cramping and discomfort on purpose—the water should be cool but never freezing. Like any other scene, negotiation and communication are crucial elements to an erotic enema. All the recommendations from chapter 5 apply to erotic enemas as well.

NOTE

1. For more information on how to do these and other BDSM activities safely, there are dozens of books on the subject, both with general overviews (like *SM 101* and *Screw the Roses, Send Me the Thorns*) and very specific topics (like *The Seductive Art of Japanese Bondage* and *The Compleat Spanker*). Find out if there is a local BDSM support group or organization in your community where you can meet other kinky people. You may want to go to a play party or a local club, where you can see people engaged in BDSM. If you see something you'd like to know more about, don't interrupt anyone's scene, but wait until they are finished and politely ask some questions. Attending BDSM workshops and demonstrations is another great way to learn safe techniques from skilled and experienced BDSM practitioners. See Resource Guide for more information.

QUOTES

Violet Blue, "Prelude to a Spanking" in *Naughty Spanking Stories From A to Z*, edited by Rachel Kramer Bussel (Point Reyes, CA: Pretty Things Press, 2004), xii.

Pauline Réage, *Story of O*, translated by Sabine d'Estree (New York: Grove Press, 1965), 83.

Butt Bondage:

Long-Term Butt Plug Wear

As I said in chapter 8, many people love the feeling of fullness you get from having a butt plug in your ass. Some people like to extend that pleasure by wearing a butt plug for a period of time. My friend Susan wears a butt plug on long traveling excursions by car and train; she says it makes the time go faster.

Other people use plugs to warm up for whatever's coming later, and like to keep them in for a while. I know another woman who likes to wear a butt plug out on a date, in order to begin foreplay over dinner at a restaurant. Through each course of the meal, she is reminded of her ass, and with every shift in her seat, she prepares her ass for bigger things to come.

Some plug lovers wear a butt plug out in public just for the hell of it. Butt plugs may hide in dark places, but they are not shy about going out on the town. Wearing a butt plug under my clothes in public can be naughty, exciting, and make running errands an ecstatic experience. It's my little secret, one the rest of the world doesn't know. When the bus hits a pothole or I shift in my seat on the subway, I get a little thrill. The next time you're on a really long line at the bank or in a stressful place like Kinko's, look around. Find the person who appears most serene, with a wide smile on his or her face, and you've discovered the one who's wearing a butt plug.

Tips for Wearing a Butt Plug

Wearing a butt plug for an extended period of time in private or out in public can be hot, fun, and sexy, and here are a few tips to make it even better. First, select a plug made of a flexible material, like rubber, jelly, or silicone; if you're going to have it in for a while, you want it to move with you and be as comfortable as possible. You should work your way up slowly. Use common sense: if you've only ever had a plug in for fifteen minutes, don't try it for four hours. Begin by wearing a butt plug for about twenty minutes; see how it feels, how you like it, what works and what doesn't. If your twenty-minute excursion goes well, try a half hour next time. Continue building up the amount of time (in reasonable increments) that you wear the plug.

You should be aware of a butt plug, but it should not feel uncomfortable or painful at all. Like anything else you put in your ass, the butt plug should be well-lubricated. You may want to consider taking it out every hour, relubing it and reinserting it. Some of you purists may consider this cheating, (if you're keeping track of how long you can keep it in) but keep in mind that the lube will be absorbed by your body eventually, and the plug may get uncomfortable. Silicone lubes won't dry up like water-based ones, but remember you cannot use them with a silicone butt plug.

Keeping It In

If you're going to be wearing a butt plug, you want to make sure it stays put, and there are many different ways to do that. Exploring different methods for keeping it in and creating something to do the job can be sexy activities you can do alone or share with a partner. Things to consider when choosing are: how you want whatever it is to look, how much time and money you want to spend on it, and how secure you want it to be.

The simplest, most affordable way to keep a plug in is to wear a tight-fitting pair of thong underwear. (If you're worried that all thongs are lacey and feminine, have no fear: they make men's thongs too.) They're easy to get, easy to put on, and, if you're wearing them out in public, no one will ever know. Depending on how they fit and the base of the plug, there could be some slippage, which is the only downside to this method.

If you're not content with a simple thong or want something more secure, you can use a butt plug harness. Harnesses come in different styles, and some can be purchased, while others are do-it-yourself. Using a harness tends to be more complicated and costly. Because wearing a harness to secure a butt plug is a form of bondage—whether done to you by you or by another person—let's first review some basic guidelines for bondage.

Bondage 101

Restraining a person or a part of their body can be an incredibly erotic experience. For the top, bondage can be an expression of power and control; for the bottom, bondage may symbolize their submission and surrender. When it comes to genital bondage or butt bondage (using a harness to keep a butt plug in the ass), it can be especially intimate.

In addition to the physical sensations of having rope or another material rubbing up against your genitals, there can be deep psychological components for the bottom: you may feel particularly submissive since such an intimate part of your body—the ass—has been stuffed and made off limits to others. Someone has tied up your private parts, and that person is the only one who can set them free. For the top, bondage can be symbolic of ownership of the bottom's ass: no one can get near it because you've blocked the entry. You may require the bottom to ask permission to go to the bathroom. However you structure the scene and the dynamic, here are some important guidelines for genital bondage:

When you're working on binding the backside, it's also going to involve the genitals, so make sure important parts—balls, urethra, clitoris, pussy—are not constricted.

Communicate with the bottom, monitor his or her breathing, body language, and circulation. If you put a bottom in bondage then send him off on errands, only do so with an experienced bondage bottom. Bondage of any kind can produce intense physical and emotional reactions, and you don't want your bottom to fall or faint without you there.

Bondage should feel snug and secure but should never be tight or constricting; it should never cut off the circulation. If you can't slip two fingers comfortably between the bondage and the person's skin, it's too tight.

As with any form of bondage, if you're going to bind a part of someone's genital area, make sure there is a fail-safe way to get out of the bondage quickly in case of an emergency, even if that means destroying the harness. Have safety scissors nearby to cut tape or rope off.

Bondage Tape Butt Plug Harness

Bondage tape is a unique invention that can be used for all your bondage needs, including creating a harness to keep a butt plug in. It's relatively inexpensive and available at sex toy stores and websites. Made of shiny PVC, bondage tape comes in different colors and one roll contains more than 60 feet of tape. It adheres to itself, but won't stick to anything else,

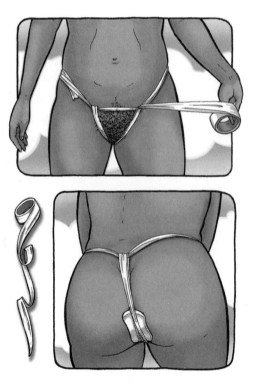

Illustration 17: Bondage Tape Butt Plug Harness

like delicate skin, hair, or furniture. Because it is exactly like tape (except it's not sticky), you don't need a lot of skill to use it. It doesn't always give a perfect snug fit and can shift around, especially when used in the genital area. If you plan to remove the plug with it on, it may be tricky to put back in. Depending on the fit, this harness may not be ideal if you're going to be doing a lot of physical activity or going out in public.

This harness is made of one continuous piece of tape; you do not need to cut the bondage tape until the very last step. Make sure you already have a well-lubed butt plug in the person's ass before you begin unrolling the tape. The tape may not lie completely flat against a person's skin; it may bunch. That's normal and not a problem as long as it's not uncomfortable.

Bondage Tape Harness Instructions

Start by holding the end of the tape on the hip bone, then wrap the roll completely around the waist once. Go past the beginning piece and stop directly over the tailbone (or just above the asscrack).

Duck the roll of tape behind the waist piece by going over the top of it, then unroll the tape straight down between the legs.

Pull the tape up between the legs in the front of the body just to the left of the pussy or cock.

Continue straight up to the front waist piece and duck the roll behind it by going over the top of it once. Unroll the tape back down between the legs following the same path the tape came from.

Duck the roll of tape behind the waist piece in back by going over the top of it.

Bring the roll straight back down between the legs, then pull the tape up between the legs in the front of the body just to the right of the pussy or cock.

Continue straight up to the front waist piece and duck the roll behind it by going over the top of it once. Unroll the tape back down between the legs following the same path the tape came from.

When you bring it back up to the waist piece in the back, before you loop it back behind you can cut it, leaving about 6 extra inches.

Take the end piece and loop it around the waist piece two times, then tuck it away.

Although bondage tape is reusable, because you've used it on and around genitals, I recommend you cut it off and throw it away.

Rope Bondage Harness

For all you rope bondage enthusiasts, putting a genital rope harness on a partner not only will keep a butt plug in his or her ass, but will give you a chance to get creative with designs and knots. If you're going to parade your bottom around at a party, you can use nylon, cotton, or hemp rope according to your taste; nylon rope is probably the most popular since it's readily available, inexpensive, and comes in many colors. Provided it's done well, a rope harness is more secure than one made of bondage tape, but it obviously takes more skill and time to put on. A rope harness can be worn underneath clothing, although if you want to completely conceal it, it takes some more creative dressing to make sure the texture of the rope and any knots aren't visible.

One of the wonderful things about a rope harness is that when the person wearing it moves, the rope rubs against both the plug in his or her

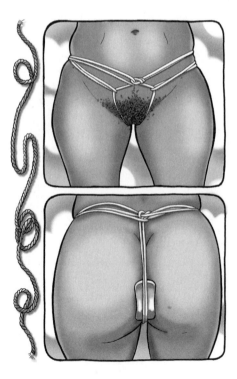

Illustration 18: Rope Bondage Butt Plug Harness

ass and the genitals; not only is a rope harness functional, it can also be very arousing. If you use rope, make sure it's not too tight and that it's soft rope that doesn't chafe or burn. Don't make complicated knots that are not easy to remove in case you have to undo them a hurry.

There are many different variations of a genital rope harness, and what follows is simply one style.[1] In this harness, the actual length of the rope will depend on the size of the body but you will most likely need 15 feet or more. Make sure you already have a well-lubed butt plug in the person's ass before you begin the rope harness.

Rope Harness Instructions

Start by folding your piece of rope in half. Hold the end that is folded on the stomach just below the belly button.

Wrap the tails around the body, bringing them back around to meet the folded end in front of the body.

Tuck the tails through the loop of the folded end and pull all the way through so the waist piece is now tight.

Tie a simple hitch by tucking the tail ends up behind the waist piece and then back down through itself (this should now enable the waist piece to remain in place hands-free).

Bring the tail ends down between the legs making sure that one piece is on either side of the cock or pussy.

Bring the rope directly up between the buttcheeks so that it presses firmly against the base of the butt plug. Loop the tail ends behind the waist piece in back once.

Take the tail piece on the left side and pull it around your waist to the right.

Take the tail piece from the right side and pull it around your waist to the left.

Bring both tail pieces back to the front of the body.

In the front of the body, loop each piece around the rope that runs between the legs and pull the tails tightly. (This will help to both tighten the harness and keep the genital area fully exposed.)

Finish the harness by tying off the ends right there or by bringing both tail pieces back around to the back of the body and tying them to each other.

When you're done, you can untie the rope harness. Because it has touched genitals and possibly bodily fluids, you should clean the rope after use; you can put it in a lingerie bag in the washing machine on the gentle cycle with a mild detergent and some bleach (color-safe bleach if the rope isn't white). Dry it on a line in long loops.

Leather Butt Plug Harness

You can purchase a leather butt plug harness at specialty leather and sex toy shops and websites (see illustrations 19 and 20). It looks very similar to a dildo harness and has a strap that runs between the buttcheeks; some designs have a piece attached to the strap that holds the base of the butt plug. Because they were designed to keep a butt plug in place, these harnesses are perfect for the job. They come in a variety of styles, and the two most popular are the plain front (ideal if the plug wearer has a pussy) or the cock ring style (for those with a cock, of course). Most come with adjustable buckles. A butt plug harness is the easiest of all harnesses to put

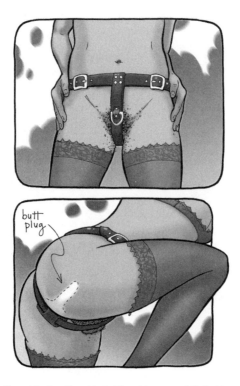

Illustration 19: Leather Butt Plug Harness (Plain Front)

on and take off by yourself since you don't need any assistance. There is also a locking style, where each buckle has a small metal ring for a small lock.

How Long Is Too Long?

So exactly how long is it safe to leave a butt plug in your ass? The literal answer is that you can leave a butt plug in for the amount of time from one bowel movement to another. This can be several hours, half a day, twenty-four hours, or more, depending on the person, so taking the question literally is not necessarily practical.

As I said before, you should work your way up to longer time increments. If you get experienced wearing butt plugs for longer periods of time, you can probably safely wear one for about six hours. Make sure to relube it periodically, and if you feel any discomfort, take it out. If your goal is to warm up your ass for something sizable there is such a thing as

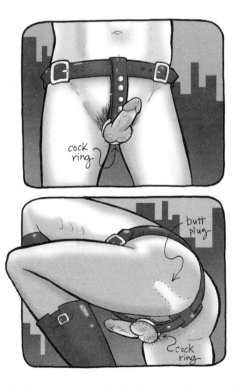

Illustration 20: Leather Butt Plug Harness (With Cock Ring)

wearing a plug for too long. If you keep it in for several hours, when it comes out, your ass may have had enough stimulation and penetration, and the evening is over.

ASK THE ANAL ADVISOR: *Harnessed for Dinner*

Q: *My partner and I are in a permanent Dominant/submissive relationship, and have been experimenting with anal sex for over two years now. We both get a lot of pleasure out of it. He likes to have me wear a locking harness to keep a butt plug in place while we go out to dinner and a movie. The trouble is, after about an hour, I need to use the restroom and must remove it. What can I do prior to "harnessing up" that will allow me to be able to wear the harness for a longer time? Should I change my diet prior to the excursion?*

A: The amount of time you can wear a butt plug depends upon your personal bathroom schedule, and everyone's particular timetable varies greatly. It sounds like you're an evening bathroom-goer, and that shortly after eating, you have to go to the bathroom. In order to prolong your butt plug wearing, I suggest that dinnertime be moved. You could eat dinner, wait to have a bowel movement, then get locked in your harness for several hours. Or perhaps you can have an outing with the butt plug in your ass that doesn't involve food, then, after the scene is over, treat yourself to a meal. If the outing must include dinner, than perhaps your top should insist that you watch *him* eat, while you're limited to water only (sorry to give him tips from my sadistic top self, but you did ask). If you're a good girl, maybe he'll feed you after you've held that butt plug in long enough!

NOTE

1. For other genital rope harnesses (as well as great information on bondage), see *The Seductive Art of Japanese Bondage* by Midori (Oakland, CA: Greenery Press, 2001), 131-134, and Jay Wiseman's *Erotic Bondage Handbook* (Oakland, CA: Greenery Press, 2000), 227-236.

15

The Art of Anal Fisting

Anal fisting, also known as handballing, is the gradual process of fitting an entire hand in the ass. The term itself can be misleading—you don't just make a fist and stick it in someone's butt. In fact, there may not be a fist at all: depending on your hand position, your fingers could be straight out or overlapped, but not curled down at all. People who like a feeling of fullness and pressure in their tushes and like to play with big toys may also dig being fisted. Fisting takes a *large* amount of everything that anal sex requires: desire, patience, relaxation, communication, trust, and, of course, lube. Fisting requires time, practice, and experience, and should not be attempted until after you have mastered the basics of anal penetration. When done safely and properly, fisting can be an incredibly intense, pleasurable experience for both partners.

It is believed that people have engaged in fisting for decades before the sexual revolution, but the recorded history of it in Western culture dates to the late sixties. In the late 1960s and 1970s, gay and bisexual men popularized the practice of anal fisting, especially in bathhouses and sex parties in cities like San Francisco, Los Angeles, and New York. Because these particular communities were doing it, teaching it, and writing about it, fisting became associated with gay men, especially leathermen, or those who practice BDSM. Anal fisting was represented in the infamous S/M hanky code by a red hanky (worn on the left by fisters, on the right by fistees), making it easier for fisting fans to find one another as well as solidifying fisting's association with BDSM.[1]

While anal fisting can be incorporated into BDSM and many consider it an intense exchange of power between two people, it does not have to involve BDSM nor is it done exclusively by people who do BDSM. Queer kinky guys pioneered anal fisting and passed on their experience and wisdom to younger generations; however, lesbians and straight men and women have also had their hands in the mix. Many of them learned about techniques and safety from gay male friends and erotica. Today, while not as common as other forms of anal eroticism, anal fisting is practiced by kinky and nonkinky people of all sexual orientations from all walks of life. In fact, the majority of folks who come to my anal fisting workshops are heterosexual men and women.

My Personal Philosophy

In 1999, I was invited to co-teach a workshop on anal fisting with a gay leatherman who has written and taught about the practice. This guy has been putting his hands in men's asses for many years, and he wrote a book on the subject. He is one of the godfathers of ass fisting. We communicated by email before the conference, and planned to meet over breakfast to discuss the class together. But, as often happens at conferences, we each got pulled in other directions, and couldn't connect before our scheduled seminar. So, we arrived at the class, each with our own outline for a fisting workshop, ready to go with the flow. Since he was older and wiser than me, I let him take the lead. He began by saying that he usually liked to smoke a joint to help him and his partner relax for a fisting scene. Wow, I thought, if there is any smoke involved in my fisting, it's probably incense, to set a sensual mood. As we continued, our differences became more and more obvious.

"Then, I like to play some deep trance music," he continued. I'm more a fan of the mellow, ethereal music of Jane Siberry.

"We'll have a glass of red wine...." Bottled water, noncarbonated, I suggested.

He brought out a large tub of Crisco, his lubricant of choice. I had my super-size bottle of thick, water-based lube with the pump attachment.

Then he moved on to poppers. Poppers, also known as amyl nitrate or butyl nitrite, are illegal (but relatively easy to obtain) drugs that you inhale. Old-school fisters swear by poppers, and consider them not just a step in their own process but one of the steps they teach. (See sidebar on fisting and poppers.)

Fisting and Poppers

POPPERS HAVE A LONG HISTORY associated with anal fisting, especially among gay men. Poppers are the popular term for various types of alkyl nitrites, including amyl nitrate, butyl nitrites, and isobutyl nitrites. Although they are illegal drugs, they are often sold as video head cleaners and are pretty easy to obtain. People inhale them to enhance sexual pleasure. Poppers cause vasodilation, a widening of blood vessels which allows increased blood flow; the body responds by speeding up the heart rate and lowering the blood pressure. When blood rich in oxygen reaches the brain, most people feel a rush which lasts for a few minutes. Poppers are not an aphrodisiac, but they do relax the sphincter muscles, which can help make anal penetration or fisting easier, which is why they are used during sex.

Poppers will cause your ass to relax temporarily, but, like any other drug, they also alter your physical and emotional state and your judgment. Poppers may lead you to go beyond what your body's limits are under normal circumstances, which could have a variety of negative consequences, both physical and emotional.

Poppers can cause skin rashes, weakness, headaches, nausea, vomiting, dizziness, feelings of falling or spinning, and loss of erection; studies show that they reduce immune system functioning for several days after use. People with compromised immune systems, heart problems, low or high blood pressure, anemia, or who are pregnant, should never use poppers. Studies show that combining poppers with other drugs (like cocaine or ecstasy) can be extremely dangerous, and using poppers with Viagra or Cialis can cause a fatal drop in blood pressure.

In terms of our theory and practice of fisting, we were night and day. The workshop could have been a disaster. But it turned out to be a true meeting of the minds and asses, a unique bridging of different perspectives, genders, and generations. I learned a great deal from him, especially about techniques and the spirituality of fisting. He is a fisting legend and he represents a community of gay leathermen who were the first to put fisting on the map; they created sex clubs and other spaces in which to do it, they wrote about it, they documented it on video. Theirs is a rich, layered history, an old-school style of fisting learned, taught, and passed down from generation to generation by gay men. That history obviously informs mine.

I learned anal fisting from dykes, and I primarily teach it to queer and straight women and straight men. I have developed my own methods for over ten years. In writing about the experience, I coined the term *New School Fister/Fistee* to describe my own personal philosophy about the subject. I believe that fisting can happen without using anything to alter our minds or bodies—I like to start from a place of being fully present and sober, since the act itself is mind- and body-altering. I'm not saying that my way is better than old school or any other way, it's just my way. As with everything else in sexuality, I encourage you to take what works for you from all different sources and experiences, and create your own path.

Preparation and Safety

Over the years, many people have asked me if they should change their diet or fast before being fisted. I don't recommend that people fast before sex of any kind, and especially not anal fisting, which can take several hours. Fasting can disrupt many of your body's natural processes, throwing everything out of whack. Besides the fact that it's never ideal to have sex while lightheaded and hungry, fasting can cause a drop in blood sugar levels, headaches, nausea, and other symptoms that will leave you feeling sick—the exact opposite of how you want to feel going into a fisting session.

So you should not refrain from eating, but should you change your eating habits? Everyone's digestive system is different, so there is no universal rule of thumb. When it comes to how *your* gastrointestinal system works, you know your ass, your bathroom schedule, and your regularity better than anyone else. However, there are a few general guidelines that apply to almost everyone. You should have a bowel movement before anal penetration in order to empty your bowels and "clear the runway" for anal play. Eating a big meal before a hot anal sex date is probably not the best idea since it's likely to stimulate digestion. In addition, if you have a particularly sensitive system, then avoid foods that are spicy or especially hard for your body to digest. You may want to also steer clear of foods with small seeds—like strawberries, raspberries, seeded bagels, and breads—since they are not digested in the upper intestinal tract. When they enter the rectum during a bowel movement, they can linger there, causing discomfort during penetration.

If you're going to be fisted, an enema is a necessity. When you're talking about fitting someone's entire hand inside your ass, hygiene is not your only concern. An enema will clean out your rectum including any stray fecal matter that could make the experience uncomfortable. Plus, since there is a greater chance of some trauma to the rectal tissue (including small tears), you want to make sure that you're as clean as you can be. You should use either an enema bag or a shower attachment (rather than the bulb syringe or bottle) for deeper cleaning. Follow the rules of enemas from chapter 5, making sure that you leave two hours or more between your enema and your fisting date to give your ass a chance to recover and regenerate that thin layer of mucous that protects the delicate rectum.

Speaking of cleanliness, since you're about to be using a whole lot of lube, it's a good idea to think about another kind of tidying-up in advance. Whether it's a bed, a bondage bench, or a sling, covering it with a towel or a disposable absorbent bed pad will protect it from unwanted spills and make post-fisting cleaning quicker and easier.[2] Also, keep a box of baby wipes nearby to catch lube spills and deal with any mess.

Contrary to some popular misconceptions, being anally fisted will not make you bleed excessively, damage your rectum, stretch out your anus, or rupture your intestines—if you do it correctly. It's important for both partners to take certain precautions to protect themselves from discomfort or injury, as well as the transmission of STDs. The risks of STD transmission outlined in chapter 6 and discussed in chapter 17 for penetration with fingers apply to fisting; however, it's much more likely that fisting could cause small tears in the rectal tissue and/or bleeding.

For the fister, it's important to wear a latex or nonlatex glove, whether or not you usually wear gloves for manual penetration. Gloves will make penetration much more comfortable for the fistee, and protect both of you should any tearing or bleeding occur during fisting. Even though you'll be wearing a glove, it is critical that your nails be short and well-filed with no sharp edges. If you have long nails (real or acrylic) that you don't want to sacrifice in order to fist someone, then remember to stuff cotton in the tips of the fingers or wrap your nails in gauze before putting on a glove. Since the average glove ends at your wrist, I suggest a longer glove for fisting. You can purchase gloves of longer lengths at medical, dental, and sex supply stores and websites. (See sidebar and Resource Guide for more information.)

Previously, some sex educators and organizations recommended wearing two gloves on one hand as a safer sex precaution (if a glove tore during sex, you were still protected by the one underneath it) or for quicker transition between orifices (you could go from ass to pussy without much interruption by simply peeling off the top glove). We know that wearing two condoms creates friction between condoms and increases the chance of a tear. Although gloves are made of a thicker form of latex or nonlatex material than condoms, there is anecdotal evidence that wearing two gloves can do the same: produce friction between the gloves that can lead to a higher chance of breakage or tearing. Stick to one glove at a time, but pay close attention, and change gloves immediately if you notice a tear or hole.

Finding Extra-Long Gloves

Standard gloves are about 9" long, extra-long gloves are 12". When looking for extra-long gloves, look for terms like "XP," "extra protection" and "high-risk use," which signify gloves that are thicker, have reinforced fingertips, are longer, or have some combination of these qualities. Here are some options and sources:

LATEX: www.cottonballs.com, www.kinkymedical.net, www.eqplus.com, www.grogans.com

NEOPRENE/CHLOROPRENE: SemperCare CRX (12"), www.cottonballs.com, www.grogans.com, www.fishersci.com

NITRILE: Kimberly Clark SafeSkin Nitrile XTRA (12"), www.fishersci.com

VINYL: Maxxim SensiCare XP, www.cottonballs.com

OTHER: Mr. S has its own line of latex gloves for fisting; they are like bondage mitts, totally enclosed with no fingers, and come in three lengths. Find them at www.mr-s-leather.com.

Keep It Real: Communication and Expectations

We're back to that C-word again, the one we return to again and again throughout this book—*communication*. Communication is a fundamental part of anal fisting, since it is an intense activity that tests the limits of our bodies and minds. Before you actually try this erotic endeavor, it's important to have an honest discussion about it. Tell your partner about your goals, expectations, and any fears you may have; get them out on the table so you can talk them through. Each partner should be clear about his or her level of experience with anal play and anal fisting. It's okay to be a novice, as long as you let your partner know in advance. If you've tried it before, discuss what worked and what didn't. The more information both of you have, the better off you'll be.

Fisting requires trust, patience, and a substantial time commitment. Even with all the skill and patience in the world, the ass can have a mind of its own, and sometimes, it just doesn't happen. Be prepared for that, so if you don't get to the whole hand-chilada, it won't surprise and disappoint you. It's important for both of you to have realistic expectations, whether it's your first try or your fourteenth. The less pressure you place on yourself and your partner, the more likely it will be to happen. But nothing will happen without verbal and nonverbal signals between you and your partner. As the fister, it's important to continually check in with your partner, make sure she/he is comfortable, and get her

> *She pushed. A ripple descended from behind her breast bone, amplified, became a wave of desperate hard contractions. Kay had a grim, fixed smile on her face. She hung on to Roxanne's thigh with one hand and kept the other one wedged firmly in her asshole.*
>
> *Her rectum opened, closed, opened wider, and Kay slid in. Her querulous asshole flattened out and disappeared. It felt as if her body had swallowed the advancing hand, sucked it in instead of struggling to repel it. Now it was folded up neatly inside her, a miracle, no pain at all, just the gift, the blessing of someone entering and pleasuring this forbidden part of her body. Kay had made this new channel, made it part of her just by touching it. Her lungs hurt. Had she been shouting?*
>
> —Pat Califia—

feedback about what you're doing. The fistee needs to direct the action, tell your partner if you need to slow down or stop, and be clear about when it's okay to proceed to the next step.

There's No Such Thing as Too Much Lube

Some fisting aficionados swear by Crisco or other oil-based or vegetable-based lubricants—like Boy Butter, Elbow Grease, ID Cream, or Men's Cream—for fisting (see sidebar on page 162 for more on Crisco). Oil-based and vegetable-based lubes are very thick and don't dry up like their water-based counterparts. Although I cautioned against them in chapter 7, if your fistee is a guy, with one orifice, and you just adore this kind of lube, then it is safe to use for fisting him. Although it's difficult to clean up, it will flush out of the rectum when he has a bowel movement. Just make sure you use nonlatex (nitrile, vinyl/polyurethane, neoprene) gloves and condoms on toys, since these lubes can break down latex. If tiny holes develop, they can cause the latex to weaken, break, and be ineffective. Sticking your hand in a can of Crisco (or a tub, which many of the lubes mentioned come in) will leave that container full of bacteria. With a clean spoon or scoop, scoop smaller amounts of lube out of the original container and into a separate one, which you can throw away after the fisting.

As I said in chapter 7, if the person you're fisting has two holes, then you should never use oil-based or vegetable-based lube in either one. Since anal fisting requires so much lube, it's likely that some of the lube will find its way to the pussy. When these lubes are introduced into the pussy, they are impossible to flush out. They become a breeding ground for vaginal infection.

My preference is for a thick water-based lube that is the consistency of hair gel. Just as these lubes are ideal for anal penetration, they work great for fisting. I prefer one that contains glycerin—brands like Astroglide Gel, Probe Thick and Rich, or J-Lube—since that ingredient helps the lube stay wet longer. If your ass is sensitive or allergic to glycerin, then try Maximus or a silicone lube.

If you're a fan of silicone lubes, then I recommend Eros Silicone Gel or Eros Cream, since Eros Original and some other brands of silicone-based lubricant are far too thin and slick to do the job for fisting; they allow too much friction, which can lead to discomfort. Keep in mind that silicone lubes are not compatible with silicone toys, so if you are planning to use silicone toys to warm up the ass before fisting, use a condom on them.

Some people like to combine two different kinds of lubes; for example, you can add a few drops of silicone lube to increase the staying power of a water-based lube while still getting the benefits of the texture of the thicker lube. If you add silicone lube to any water-based lube, then consider it a silicone lube and follow guidelines about not using it on silicone toys without a condom. Whatever lube you choose, never use one that contains nonoxynol-9, as it is more likely to irritate the rectal tissue and make fisting uncomfortable or painful.

You want whatever it is you're using to penetrate someone's ass—your fingers, a toy, your cock—to be coated in lube. Each time you introduce another finger, or readjust, add more lube. Be generous and remember that more lube equals more comfort and easier penetration for the fistee. In order to prepare the ass for what's to come, I also like to make sure I get lube way up inside the rectum. Once you're in the heat of the fisting, you don't want to have to slide your hand all the way out, relube, then work on getting all the way back in again. This not only breaks the momentum, but it can stress the sphincter muscles as well.

There are several tools I use to shoot lube up someone's ass so it's waiting for me when I finally get my whole hand (or almost my whole hand) inside. The Lube Shooter is a disposable plastic syringe (with a flared base) that was designed for this very purpose. Simply remove the plunger, fill the syringe with lube, and replace the plunger. Before you put it in someone's ass, push the plunger down a little to begin the flow of lube and let any air out. Lube the plastic tip of the syringe and gently insert it into the ass. Push the plunger down gently to release the lube. You can refill it and repeat. When you're done, throw it away. Astroglide makes an even more convenient product called the Astroglide Shooter. It's a soft plastic 5 ml tube of lube with a long neck for easy insertion. You don't need to fill these and they can be more comfortable for some people since they are made of softer plastic than the Lube Shooter. Twist off the tab, lube the tip, and slide it in. You can also use disposable plastic irrigation syringes that come in different sizes (commonly 50, 60, or 100 ml) and are available at medical supply stores and some specialty sex product websites.

If you like the look of metal, are into medical toys, or simply want to use something that looks a lot more menacing than a small plastic syringe, then I recommend a stainless steel syringe—often called an enema syringe or a lube syringe—which you can find on medical fetish and other specialty sex product websites. It holds a lot more lube than the plastic ones and has a decidedly more daring aesthetic. Made of polished metal, it comes with two interchangeable tips (pointy and rounded) and is available in several different sizes; the most common are 100 cubic centimeters (cc) and 200 cc (which are equivalent to 100 ml and 200 ml). The 200-cc syringe is the size of a large, thick dildo, so it should only be used on very experienced bottoms. To use it, pull back the plunger, then unscrew the top and fill the body with lube. Replace the top, then push the plunger down a little to begin the flow of lube and let any air out *before you insert it*. Then lube the tip, carefully insert it into the ass, and push the plunger down. To clean the syringe, take it apart, and wash it gently with warm water and antibacterial soap. Since this toy has a bunch of nooks and crevices, I like to go one step further and soak it for a few minutes in a diluted bleach solution (10 parts water, 1 part bleach). Make sure you dry all the parts completely, since if left damp, they can rust. (See Resource Guide for where to purchase these items.)

The Power of Crisco

ASK ANY GAY LEATHERMAN (and some women) of a certain generation what the best fisting lube is, and their answer will be the same: Crisco. Yes, *that* Crisco. It's not just for baking cookies anymore! I even recommended Crisco in the first edition of this book. I have since had a lot more experience with fisting, and now I no longer recommend it. I don't caution against it if the person being fisted is male, because it's ultimately safe. But for female-bodied people and others, I think there are much better products for the job. Nonetheless, there are people out there who will forever swear by it. I think people have a very emotional relationship to Crisco. For them, it conjures images of the first time they ever went to a fisting club, like the Catacombs in San Francisco in the seventies, and discovered a community of men doing what they loved to do. Crisco has cultural significance that is unmatched; it is synonymous with an era of asses up in slings, underground clubs, red hankies, and an alternative, sex-radical world still on the fringes of society.

Positions for Fisting

As with other anal activities, there are a number of different positions, each with its own particular benefits, for anal fisting. The ideal position for fisting is one that will allow easy ass access and give both fister and fistee the comfort to be there for an extended period of time. For doing it on a bed, I like to use firm pillows or Liberator Shapes, a unique brand of firm, supportive shapes that help to angle the body better for different kinds of penetration and stimulation. An overstuffed, comfortable chair can offer good back support and comfort for the fistee, and the fister can kneel or sit on a pillow in front of the chair. The slings and swings discussed in chapter 11 are also great for anal fisting. Fistees should position themselves in a sling or swing so that all parts of their bodies feel supported and nothing is constricted. Fisters can sit or stand between the fistee's legs; you should adjust the height of the sling so that you don't have to bend or slouch.

Whether you end up in a sling or on the ol' Sealy Posturpedic, here are some examples of anal fisting positions. All the pros and cons discussed in chapter 11 about positions for anal penetration apply to these as well.

MISSIONARY WITH KNEES UP: Fistee on her/his back with fister sitting or kneeling between fistee's legs. To insure full access to the back door, prop up the butt (in order to tip the hips up and back slightly) with a firm pillow or the Liberator Shapes wedge and have your partner spread her/his legs with knees bent.

LEGS OVER SHOULDERS: Fistee on her/his back with fister sitting or kneeling between fistee's legs. Fistee folds legs so knees touch chest or legs flip up and over shoulders. This configuration only works if the fistee can stay in it for a while without discomfort.

MISSIONARY ON THE EDGE: Fistee on her/his back at the edge of the bed (or a massage table, a bondage table, a spanking bench, or a comfortable stuffed chair) with fister between fistee's legs, either standing or sitting in a chair of the appropriate height.

DOGGIE-STYLE/ON ALL FOURS: Fistee on hands and knees, fister kneels behind (if on the bed) or stands behind (if using edge of the bed or other furniture).

DOGGIE-STYLE/HEAD DOWN: Same as Doggie-Style/On All Fours, except fistee's head and shoulders are down.

DOGGIE/BENT OVER FURNITURE: Fistee bent over a bed, couch, table with fister standing behind.

IN A SLING OR SWING.

Work Your Way In

As you are preparing to fist someone, one of your most important goals should be to get his or her ass warmed-up, relaxed, open, and ready *without wearing it out*. You have to walk a fine line between playing with an ass enough to get it wanting more and playing with it *too* much. If you cross that line, the ass is tired, sore, and done. So, you've got to figure out what kinds of stimulation work for your particular fistee's butt. Does she need to have vaginal penetration, clitoral stimulation, and her first orgasm of the night in order to begin? For multiorgasmic people, coming can relax their body, take the edge off, and allow them to begin the process of opening up. Maybe he wants a slow, sensual blow job with his favorite plug nestled in his ass. Genital stimulation sends blood rushing to the entire genital region, including the anal area, and the butt plug will help his ass start to relax. Remember that desire and arousal are unique to the individual, so discover what works for you (or your partner)—what gets you to that place where you are revved up and ready—and do that.

For some folks, fisting is all about the hand. All anal stimulation comes from the fingers, beginning with one, then two, then three, four, five, and, hopefully, past the widest part, until the whole hand fits inside. If you take this approach, your fingers do not need to go straight in; you can explore different finger positions as you cross one finger on top of the other. Don't forget to curve your fingers toward the G-spot or the prostate for extra stimulation. When you first add another finger (accompanied by more lube, of course), don't go all the way inside. Go just past the first knuckle, and stay still until the body gets used to the addition. Then carefully slide farther inside. If you are the recipient, let your partner know when you're ready for another finger; you should feel open and aroused, and the penetration will feel comfortable and pleasurable. Everyone's fingers and hands are different sizes, and, as a general rule, men's hands are bigger than women's hands. Use these tips as a guideline, but if you have large fingers, keep in mind that your process may be slower as a result. You can switch from fingers to a dildo or vibrator (as long as it has a flared base) to create a different sensation.

If you find that a lot of in-and-out penetration with fingers or dildos puts too much stress on the sphincter muscles and wears out the ass too quickly, butt plugs are the perfect solution. I like to use butt plugs for warm-up as an alternative to other kinds of stimulation because they simultaneously create a pleasurable sensation and help the ass begin to open up. Start with a well-lubed small butt plug, and have your fistee wear it for about twenty minutes to a half hour. During that time, you can concentrate on other things—dirty talk, cock and ball play, vaginal penetration, clit stimulation, tit torture, whatever. While you're busy entertaining your partner (and yourself), the butt plug is working its magic: helping the ass adjust to having something inside it and relax in the process. Take the toy out carefully, and slip a finger or two inside to gauge how aroused and relaxed the ass is. Ideally, penetration will feel easy. Move on to a medium-size plug, and keep that in for about a half hour as you continue with other kinds of stimulation. When you've both agreed that the ass is ready for more, insert a large plug (I recommend one with a diameter of two inches or more), which the fistee can wear for up to an hour. (Review the previous chapter for long-term butt plug wear information.)

Four Fingers and Beyond

After the large butt plug is removed, I like to start penetration with three or four fingers. That may sound extreme, but remember that the person's ass has had a butt plug in it for a couple of hours by now. Move from three to four fingers, taking care to add more lube and go as slow as you need to. However you get to four fingers, this is the point where you should decide whether to continue or stop genital stimulation. Some people need stimulation to have anything in their ass feel pleasurable, and four or five

---

Tips for Fisters

File your nails and wear a well-fitting latex or nonlatex glove.

Talk to your partner before and during the fisting.

Use butt plugs that graduate in size for warm-up.

Always add lube to your hand or toy as you progress.

Experiment with different hand positions.

If your fisting hand starts to get tired, grasp the wrist with your other hand to steady it, support it, and even help guide it in.

---

fingers is no exception. For that reason, keep working her clit or his cock while you've got your fingers inside. For other people, while genital stimulation may feel great, it also causes their sphincter muscles to contract. To the fister, these contractions can feel like a vice clamping down on your fingers and the tightness can prevent you from getting any farther. One solution is for the fistee to concentrate on relaxing the sphincters by taking deep breaths and bearing down. If one becomes aware of the contractions, one may be able to lessen them. If that doesn't work, it may be time to back off of genital stimulation altogether and concentrate solely on the anal penetration. As discussed in chapter 12, this may also be the point when a man who is being fisted loses his erection.

At the four-finger mark, you should discover which finger and hand positions work best for the specific butt you're working over. Here are some examples:

PALM UP: With the receptive partner on his/her back, the fister's hand is palm up with middle and ring finger flat and straight, index finger and pinky pointed inward. The thumb can rest on top of the base of the index finger; this creates a natural funnel for lube to run down and into ass. You can manipulate the G-spot or the prostate with the tips of the fingers. As you get farther inside, you'll want to tuck the thumb closer to the center of the hand (between index finger and pinky) to tighten up the size of the hand.

PALM DOWN: Identical to Palm Up, but used when the fistee is in doggie-style position. The fister's hand is reversed so the palm is down (toward the front of the fistee's body). You lose the funneling ability to gravity, but can still hit the G-spot or the prostate with the tips of the fingers.

PALM UP OR PALM DOWN WITH CURL: This hand position is similar to Palm Up or Palm Down, except the fingers spread out and curl down and the thumb is tucked under them to make a fist.

HANDSHAKE: Start with the receptive partner on his/her back, and put your hand out like you're about to shake someone else's hand. Leave the middle and ring finger flat and straight, and bring the index finger and pinky pointed inward and on top of the other two fingers. Bring the thumb to the middle of the hand. Once inside, you can bend your thumb slightly and use the thumb knuckles to stimulate the G-spot or the prostate. You can duplicate this hand position when your partner is on his or her hands and knees, except without the benefit of the thumb-knuckle trick.

HANDSHAKE WITH CURL: Begin with the Palm Up with Curl position, then rotate your wrist 90 degrees to the left.

In the beginning, feel free to explore many different hand positions. I like to let someone's ass tell me which position will work the best. In other words, in order to discover the ideal placement of the hand, assess the internal geography of the ass. How pronounced is the curve of the rectum? Is there more room on the front wall or the back wall? Can you find extra space if you move slightly to the left or the right? Once you get to four fingers, you should commit to one hand position since a major shift at that stage isn't a good idea.

Moving from four fingers to five should be relatively easy, since the pinky is the smallest of the bunch. Then comes the toughest challenge: getting the widest part of the hand inside. This is the place that's the most difficult to get past, the place where most people get "stuck." In my experience, at this stage of the game, there is room inside the rectum, which you'll recall can expand a great deal during anal play. However, the fister has got to contend with the gatekeepers—the anal opening, the sphincter muscles, and the anal canal—which comprise the narrowest, tightest part of the butt's anatomy. You want to apply enough gentle pressure to let the muscles know you're there and be able to gauge the amount of resistance, but you never want to force your way in. It's a delicate dance of give and take, during which you and your partner need to constantly communicate. When or if you do feel resistance or a tightening of the muscles, stay where you are and give the muscles a chance to get used to the feeling.

Each person likes to use a different method for entry. Some people like to move with a slow, constant pressure. Others use a gentle twisting motion to work their way inside. Some let the receiver draw the hand inside or go slowly in and out as you would with a penis or dildo (although the sucking motion that can happen with toys or a few fingers isn't going to happen with a whole hand). At this point, I like to pace my breathing to match the inhales and exhales of the person I am fisting. It helps ground us, connect us, and get us in sync. It also helps both of us focus on the task and experience at hand. Try inching your way in on the exhales. For the fistee, this is when relaxation is crucial. Take a deep breath—a really deep breath. Then another. Concentrate on feeling the breath move through your body. If you've been "working out" the sphincters, their toned elasticity will reward you as the widest part of your partner's hand is able to slip through the snug ring and past it into the more spacious rectum.

Once You're In

The physical and emotional rush that both partners will feel when the entire hand slips inside is incredibly intense. Take a moment, take a deep breath, and stay exactly where you are. Fister, let your hand get used to the new feeling of being entirely encased. You may feel the sphincters clamp down around your wrist; don't panic, they should relax after a few minutes. Fistee, keep breathing. Adjust to the sensation of newfound fullness.

Once the hand is all the way in, you've got a few options. Some fistees (especially novices) will not be able to tolerate having an entire hand in their ass for more than a few minutes. As the receiver, you are in control of the action. It's critical that you pay attention to your body, know your limits, and communicate with your partner. Do not push yourself to do something if your body isn't ready. Rest and take a break if you need one. If you're done, say you're done.

If you want to continue, so should your communication. As the fistee, you call the shots. Your partner will take all cues from you, and so you need to be aware of your desires, your needs, and the sensations you are feeling. Maybe you want your partner's hand to stay exactly where it is while she or he continues (or reintroduces) genital stimulation. Maybe you want to stimulate yourself or use a vibrator. If you want your partner's hand to move a little farther inside, then remain still, say so, and guide her or him.

Fisters, if your fistee asks for some movement, proceed slowly and gently. All your movements should be understated unless directed otherwise. Begin with a subtle in-and-out motion, and see how your partner responds. Depending on your hand position, use fingertips or knuckles to stimulate the G-spot or the prostate. I've had fistees tell me that the tiniest movements of my hand feel like deep pushes in the sensitive rectum. I've also fisted people who like a powerful, in-and-out thrusting motion. And, of course, there are plenty of folks' desires that fall in between these two ends of the sensation spectrum. Be mindful that fisting may or may not build up to and conclude with an orgasm. For some people, the sensation created by a fist is incredibly unique, but not orgasmic. For others, it's a case of *too much* stimulation, and their bodies may feel too overwhelmed to come. If an orgasm is in the cards for you, congratulations! The contractions an orgasm will produce can create a lot of tension around the hand, so fisters should ride the wave with their partners, then gently and slowly extract their hand. Coming out is easier than going in, however it may cause some discomfort for the fistee, especially as the widest part of the hand slips through those sphincters. I like to rub some lube around the anal opening and my wrist to help make the exit as smooth as possible.

Tips for Fistees

If you have a sensitive stomach, eat mild foods before your fisting date.

After your enema, give yourself at least two hours before anal play begins.

Practice relaxation techniques like deep breathing and meditation or whatever helps you relax.

Find a position that you'll be able to sustain comfortably for several hours.

If your partner can't reach your genitals during penetration, stimulate them yourself with your hand or a vibrator.

Ask the Anal Advisor: *Fisting Yourself*

Q: *I really want to be able to fist myself! I need your advice on how I can do it. I can fit four fingers up there, but cannot get past the knuckles at the base of the fingers. Can you help me?*

A: I don't know many folks besides gay porn stars who can fist themselves. More power to you for getting as far as you have already, and, of course, for wanting even more! It seems to me that fisting yourself is all about body position and flexibility. You are ahead of the game if you've already gotten four fingers inside. You didn't mention the position that you've been in, but I think that being on all fours or even squatting would work best. Now, if you find that you just can't make it happen, remember that there are some cool dildos on the market which are made to look just like a curled fist. You can find them in gay leather shops and catalogs usually. Having an "extra fist" means you can experiment with lots of different positions, and you aren't limited by the size of your own hand.

Aftercare

Anal fisting shouldn't hurt, and if you experience pain, you should slow down, back off, or stop altogether. If you don't, you are more likely to cause some kind of trauma to the delicate rectal tissue, which can lead to discomfort, pain, and damage to your ass. To keep your ass happy and healthy, practice common sense, and don't over do it. The better you treat it, the more you'll be able to fist it!

That said, even those who exercise care and caution may be left the next day with a butt that's out of sorts. You may experience soreness, mild bleeding, cramping, gas, or irregular bowel movements. Don't worry, these symptoms are common after such an intense, extensive anal play activity. You may feel like having another enema in order to clean out or soothe your ass, but don't. Your system has been worked over, and an enema will only irritate your rectum, especially if there are minute abrasions. Give your ass a rest from anal play, and use witch hazel wipes to relieve any external irritation.[3] Your ass should right itself within twenty-four hours. As always, use common sense: if you are bleeding, experiencing severe pain, have a fever, or feel very sick, go see a doctor immediately. If you've listened to your body, and your partner has listened to you, then besides some minor soreness, anal fisting will leave you satisfied and happily exhausted.

Fisting is truly an erotic journey of the body, mind, and spirit. Although I have covered many tips and techniques throughout this section of the book, I want to admit an important point: often, successful fisting is 20 percent experience and skill and 80 percent frame of mind. By frame of mind, I mean that the fistee has to be in a mental state that allows them to wrap their head around the notion of wrapping their ass around a hand—without anxiety, reservation, or fear. What gets someone into such a headspace? Well, that's the million-dollar question. The answer: it depends on the person. Everyone is unique, and the one thing or combination of things that will lead a person to surrender to the fist is not something I can teach you. It may be a Dominant/submissive dynamic, a hot flogging scene, the right butt plug, intense clitoral stimulation, or something else entirely. Find what it is, and you're more than halfway there.

I call this chapter The Art of Anal Fisting because I truly believe that there is an art and a beauty to this sexual experience that some may see as radical or extreme. For me, anal fisting is an expression of love, lust, faith, and trust. Having your entire hand inside someone, or having someone's hand inside you, is like no other feeling in the world. When I do it, I feel alive, amazed, even high, and deeply connected to my body and my partner.

NOTES

1. The hanky code was a signaling system that originated in the gay male leather community, but has been adopted by kinky people of all sexual orientations. A handkerchief worn in the left pocket indicates the wearer is a top or wants to give a particular activity; a hanky worn on the right means the wearer is a bottom or wants to receive that activity. Different hanky colors represent different activities like fisting, bondage, heavy S/M, et cetera. For my adapted version of the hanky code, see www.puckerup.com/bdsm_&_fetish/hanky_code_for_heteros/.

2. Disposable absorbent bed pads, sometimes referred to as "chucks," are square or rectangular sheets made of waterproof plastic on one side, and absorbent material on the other. They were designed for use with incontinent people, to protect beds and furniture. You can find them at most drugstores in the same aisle as incontinence products.

3. Witch hazel wipes are sold in drugstores as "medicated hemorrhoidal wipes" from brands like Preparation H and Tucks. I like the Preparation H wipes better because they are about twice the size. Many drugstores also carry the generic or in-store brand, which contains the exact same ingredients but is a lot cheaper. While they are marketed for hemorrhoid relief, they are also great at soothing itchy, irritated, sore, or simply overworked asses. They are cool, soothing, and almost immediately calming for an itchy, sore, or irritated butthole. They are also great on a well-used pussy!

QUOTE

Pat Califia, "The Calyx of Isis" in *Macho Sluts* (Los Angeles: Alyson Publications, 1988), 135.

CHAPTER 16

Troubleshooting:
Common Issues and Problems

Since 1997, I have answered questions from people all over the world via email or in person at my workshops on a variety of issues and problems related to anal play. Here are some of the most common.

Is it safe to have anal sex when I am pregnant?

Throughout your pregnancy, penetration with fingers (both vaginal and anal) is safe; penetration with a cock or dildo is safe in low-risk pregnancies. Your mate should definitely avoid deep thrusting and really hard slamming of any kind. One of the challenges of sex during pregnancy is finding comfortable positions, but that takes just a little bit of experimentation. Hemorrhoids are very common during pregnancy, so your ass may be too irritated for anal play to be enjoyable. Hygiene is really important, since yeast or bacterial infections in the vagina can be more uncomfortable and harder to treat when you are pregnant. It's especially important to prevent bacteria from the ass from transferring to the vagina, so make sure anything that goes inside you is clean and never go directly from ass to vagina. If you feel any discomfort during any sexual activity, stop at once. Talk to your obstetrician or midwife for more specific information.

ASK THE ANAL ADVISOR: *Burned Butt*

Q: *I've had a black vinyl butt plug for two years and I think that a chemical film or something has developed on the surface that makes it burn when I insert it into my girlfriend's ass. Would an automotive-type vinyl restorer make my butt toys last longer?*

A: Latex rubber, jelly rubber, and vinyl sex toys are inexpensive for a reason: they do not last forever. I recommend that folks replace toys made of these materials after twelve months for the exact reason you report: the material starts to break down, and often causes stinging, burning, itching, and other discomfort when used. No, a vinyl restorer sold in automotive supply stories is not a good idea; not only will it not help stop the toy from deteriorating, but you do not want any product like that (or traces of it) in your ass! Throw the toy out and buy a new one, or, for your next purchase, try a higher quality silicone toy. Silicone can be much more pricey, but it's also a lot more resilient. My silicone toys have lasted for many years, and some brands even come with lifetime guarantees.

Every time I try to penetrate my wife's ass, I lose my erection. I think it takes me such a long time to try and position my dick that I just lose my excitement. I don't have this problem when we have vaginal sex.

The bottom line is that you need to have a rock-hard cock to get it into someone's ass. Since you have no erectile issues during vaginal sex, your problem is probably not physical but psychological. My initial question for you is, do you have any fears about fucking your wife in the ass? Some men are anxious about hurting their partners. Somewhere in the back of your mind, you may be afraid you'll cause her pain, or perhaps a past lover has told you that you hurt her. If you think you might have this fear, reassure yourself and your wife that you're going to warm her up, use lots of lube, and go slow, so that it won't hurt. Speaking of going slow, it sounds like that may also be part of your problem. You wrote about how much time it takes to get in position, and you may be losing the momentum of the moment. If that is the case, perhaps your wife can stroke your cock as you're maneuvering it or talk dirty to you to keep the fantasy and the anticipation going while you get ready.

Any toy I put in my ass seems too long. It feels almost like the dick or the toy is hitting something inside of me, and it hurts.

The rectum is not a straight tube. It has a gentle curve, first tipping forward toward the front of the body, then back, then forward again. Everyone's curves are different, and some are more pronounced than others. If you stick anything straight inside the rectum, you can wind up hitting the rectal wall. Toys made of flexible materials are more comfortable and bend easier with your curves; if a toy itself is curved, the curve should be aimed toward the front of the body. All that said, you can also have a short rectum. Experiment with different toys, and have your partner experiment with different positions and angles. Go with what works.

When my husband penetrates my ass, initially it's fine, but then it feels like he's hitting some second ring of muscle. Once he gets all the way inside, it's fine, but when we start moving, he slips out past that ring again, and it hurts when he comes back through it.

There are two sets of sphincter muscles, the external sphincters and the internal sphincters. For some people, these two rings of muscles are quite close together, but for others, they are farther apart. Both sets of muscles need to relax completely in order for anal penetration to be comfortable and pleasurable. They are like the gatekeepers to the ass. Concentrate on relaxing; it's critical to your enjoyment. Penetration can be painful if you are nervous or tense. You and your husband can also experiment with different positions; you can change the angle of insertion, the depth of penetration, and the point at which he's hitting that inner sphincter. He also can try more shallow thrusts, so that he doesn't consistently pull out too far, which is obviously painful for you. I think your problem can be solved with some creativity in positions.

My girlfriend and I have tried anal sex multiple times, but she doesn't like it unless I rub her clit. As soon as I stop rubbing it, she says it's very painful and wants to stop. We only do it lying on our sides, facing the same direction. She claims that doggie-style hurts too much from our one time of trying it. I am an anal addict denied!

It fascinates me that you consider yourself an "anal addict denied," because you are, in fact, having anal sex—just not necessarily in the exact way you want to be. If your wife doesn't like it doggie-style, that's most likely because that position offers the deepest penetration, and it obviously doesn't work for her; fucking her in the spooning position may mean less deep thrusting for you, but a lot more comfort for her. If you're simply dying to do it to her doggie-style, then I suggest more shallow strokes. See if that feels better to her. As for your problem that she doesn't like anal unless you rub her clit, well, what exactly is the problem? Rub her clit! I know lots of women who can't take anything in their ass without something working their clit; it helps them relax, get aroused, and it just feels great. If rubbing her clit is difficult because of your body position, then let your wife work her own clit while you concentrate on her ass; that way, it's a win-win situation.

My boyfriend's dick is very big and thick. He says he will go slow, but he never listens to himself. I'm afraid that if we have anal sex, just before he's getting ready to come, he will start to do it harder and hurt me.

First, I recommend you really focus on extended foreplay before your boyfriend even attempts penetration with his dick. Have him go down on you, stimulate your clitoris, use a vibrator—whatever it takes to get you really turned on. You also need to warm up your ass with something smaller than your boyfriend's dick, like his fingers or a smaller dildo or vibrator. Make sure you are in the driver's seat. You call the shots about how hard, how deep, how fast. Talk to your boyfriend and make sure he knows when something feels really good and when it does not. Some men need some very quick hard thrusts in order to orgasm. It sounds like that may be the case with your guy. If he simply can't slow down or if he does slow down, he can't come, then I suggest this: when he's ready to shoot, have him pull out. Then you can give him a hand job, he can touch himself, or he can thrust against you but not inside you.

My boyfriend and I have been exploring anal sex together, and it's been really great. But if I come before he does, it hurts for him to continue thrusting. It's like I want his cock out of me right that very minute.

Every woman should be so lucky to have your problem! Your ass, like your pussy, contracts during orgasm. After you climax, all the blood that rushed to your genital area disperses, and your ass returns to its nonaroused state (and doesn't want a cock inside it). Well, I've had firsthand experience with your particular dilemma; I too sometimes come first and find it difficult to go on. So, what can you do? You can try to delay your orgasm until after his climax. That way, you extend your pleasure for even longer, and don't have any discomfort. Or after you come, have him slow down his movement or even stop thrusting, but still stay in your ass. Take a few minutes to recover from your mind-blowing orgasm, then concentrate on relaxing your ass by taking lots of deep breaths. To extend your arousal, play with your pussy and clit, and have him slowly resume his in-and-out movements. Continue to breathe deeply, work your clit, and relax your ass. As he pumps your ass, talk to him and let him know how it feels. Hopefully, you can have a second orgasm in the process!

Ask the Anal Advisor: *Burning Sensation*

Q: *I've taken things in my ass before, like my own fingers and a medium-sized butt plug. When my lover inserted a lubed, gloved finger into my butt, I felt an intense burning sensation. We used Eros lube and a latex glove. I know I don't have a latex allergy because I work as an EMT and use latex gloves every day. Have you ever encountered a similar situation? If so, what was the problem, and how did it get fixed?*

A: Have you considered that you may have had an allergic reaction to the lube? Different people have different sensitivities to lubricants; you may want to try a water-based lubricant (Eros is silicone-based) to see if it makes a difference. If it's not the lube, it may be some kind of anal ailment. Hemorrhoids, anal fissures, even a minute tear in the delicate lining of the rectum can cause itching, irritation, burning, or pain. In that case, give your ass a vacation from butt play for about a week, then try again. There's one other possible explanation: your ass just didn't want to be fucked that night and the "burning" was a form of pain. In other words, sometimes we register pain in different ways: as soreness, as tightness, and, in some cases, as burning. Remember that our butts can be finicky, and we need to respect them. There are times when no matter how much you've prepared, no matter how much warm-up, no matter how much you want it, your ass just won't cooperate. If your burning persists, you should see a physician.

After an anal play session, I get abdominal cramps.

Cramping after anal sex is not unusual. I have a few suggestions. First, don't fuck on a full stomach. If your body is trying to digest a big meal, then stimulation in the rectum could confuse the natural bowel processes. Similarly, just like you shouldn't drink gallons of water before you work out your abdominal muscles at the gym, the same holds true for getting fucked in the ass. Second, consider using a shorter dildo or, if it's your partner's cock, not going all the way in. The longer the cock, the closer it gets to the lower colon, which for some people may disrupt colonic activity and cause cramps. Finally, if your partner thrusts in and out of you, air can be pushed inside your rectum and travel upward in the body, giving you cramps. If the cramping persists, consult a physician; you may be suffering from a gastrointestinal problem.

Several times right after anal sex, my wife has gotten a brutal headache. She suffers from the occasional non-sex-related migraine, but her post-anal sex headaches are worse by far.

If your wife is having a headache worse than a migraine, it must be extremely painful and debilitating. At first glance, the problem seems completely unrelated to anal sex; however, it's too much of a coincidence since it's happened several times. Stress and tension can often cause a severe headache, so I have a few theories. First, while you're fucking her in the ass, she may be in a position that's putting undue strain on her neck. I know that sometimes I end up in weird positions—especially when I have my ass in the air and my head down—while buttfucking. Afterward, I often feel pain in my neck, and that pain could lead to a headache. Make sure her head and neck have plenty of support.

My second theory has to do with her breathing patterns during sex. Many people (me included!) often take very shallow breaths when we get aroused on our way to orgasm—it's a natural instinct. Masturbation guru Dr. Betty Dodson scolded me once that if I am not taking deep breaths, then the blood cannot properly circulate throughout my body during sex. Shallow breaths may cause a quick high, but deep breaths ensure that the blood is flowing and the high people often feel during sex will last throughout the act. If your wife is taking quick breaths, or even holding her breath at some points, she could be depriving her brain of oxygen. This repeated deprivation could cause an intense headache, especially if she's susceptible to headaches in the first place. It's a good idea for her to talk to her physician about the problem.

Sometimes, after anal sex, if we both have done a lot of thrusting, my wife says her ass feels numb or throbs. She says it is not pain, just discomfort. If we just do a short session (like five minutes of pumping) she does not have this feeling.

Feeling numb and throbbing are two very different sensations in my book, so I am going to address them separately. Because the ass is full of nerve endings and thus very sensitive, your wife should never have a numb feeling; indeed, most people say it's quite the opposite: their nerves are electrified. If the numbing sensation continues, I would suggest she consult a physician, because she may have a circulatory problem. As for the throbbing, once the area is engorged and it's been vigorously stimulated through repeated thrusting, throbbing seems like a natural response. You've worked her ass over well, and it's responding! As long as the throbbing subsides and she doesn't feel any pain, then I'd say you're doing a good job.

When I pulled a vibrating butt plug out of my girlfriend's ass after a short play session, a large amount of mucouslike substance came out of her ass as well.

When stuff that we don't recognize comes out of our asses it can be alarming, so I understand your concern completely. Rest assured, you are fine. The rectum is lined with a thin layer of mucous that helps to protect it. When we put toys inside our butts, some of that mucous can cling to the toy, and even mix with lubricant, which sounds like what happened to you. The rectum naturally regenerates the mucous, so your ass will return to normal. Then you can stick more things in it!

I have my penis pierced with an ampallang piercing—a horizontal piercing through the head. I'm afraid I'll get stuck in her ass if I don't pull out before ejaculation.

How big is the jewelry? If it is bigger than about 10 gauge, that would be cause for concern. I have not heard of people with average-size ampallang piercings getting stuck. Although I do think you should be concerned that your piercing may tear the delicate tissue that lines the rectum or cause your partner pain. I recommend you wear a condom to prevent possible injury or discomfort. A penis piercing with average-size jewelry should not interfere with the safe use of condoms. Use a condom with a receptacle end to fit comfortably over the jewelry, and lubricate the inside of the condom as well as the jewelry itself to reduce friction. By the way, how old is your piercing? Most piercers recommend an initial healing time of 8–10 weeks; an ampallang piercing will be fully healed at 6–12 months. If your piercing is less than 10 weeks old, give it more time to heal before you engage in anal penetration.

I want to piss in my partner's ass while fucking her.

You need a dependable erection in order to penetrate her ass, and once you're super hard, you may not be able to pee; some men can't stay that hard and let it flow. If your dick can stand up and piss, then you've got to consider the safer sex issues. As far as bodily fluids go, urine is nearly, but not completely, sterile. Peeing in your sweetheart's butt is mostly safe for you unless you have any cuts or open sores on your cock. She may want to know that she can get chlamydia, gonorrhea, hepatitis B, cytomegalovirus (CMV), or genital herpes, if these viruses are present in your piss. Unfortunately, there is no research on the transmission of HIV through urine; however, we know that HIV can be present in urine or in urine that contains a small amount of blood. If the two of you have been tested for all these diseases and are monogamous, then you should be all right. Remember that whatever you put in a rectum will be instantaneously absorbed into the bloodstream, so she may end up with an upset stomach. You might also consider peeing outside of her ass, which is even safer and still plenty of fun.

Anal Health, Anal Ailments, and STDs

Anal Health

A healthy ass is a happy ass, and a happy ass is one ready to receive anal pleasure. There are a few simple but important things you can do to keep your butt in tip-top shape, and most of them are commonsense tips for living a healthy life. Good bathroom habits are critical to your anal health, including proper hygiene and always wiping front to back. Listen to your body when it sends the signal that it's time for a bowel movement; holding it in can only lead to problems. Drink plenty of water (8–10 full glasses are recommended) and eat a balanced, fiber-rich diet. Fruits, green leafy vegetables, whole grain breads and cereals, and bran are good sources of fiber. Exercising and reducing your stress level both have positive benefits for your overall health, as well as the health of your butt. During sex, treat your behind with love and respect, follow the steps outlined in this book, and always stop any activity if it hurts. All of these things will contribute to the good health of your ass.

It's equally important to arm yourself with information about anal maladies and sexually transmitted diseases (STDs, also known as sexually transmitted infections or STIs) so you can be aware when something may be wrong. The most important thing you can do is pay attention to your body. If you experience a change in bowel movements, any of the symptoms discussed in this chapter, or anything out of the ordinary, you should see a health care professional immediately. The information in this chapter should be used only as a guideline and not a substitute for the advice of a doctor.

It is also crucial that you have a doctor with whom you feel absolutely comfortable. Lots of people feel embarrassed talking about certain health concerns, especially when it comes to their asses. Talk honestly about your symptoms as well as your anal sex practices so your health care provider has all the information he or she needs to make a proper diagnosis. This may not be the sexiest chapter in the book, but it's a necessary one. Plus, fucking without anxiety *is* sexy.

Sexually Transmitted Diseases

Part of maintaining our anal health is learning about sexually transmitted diseases and taking proper precautions to protect ourselves and our partners. In this section, I cover the most common STDs in America, their symptoms, and their treatments. Since this book is primarily concerned with anal sex and health, I specifically discuss STDs that can be transmitted through anal sex and how the STDs affect your anus and rectum. You should never attempt to self-diagnose an STD; if you suspect you may have one, see a doctor as soon as possible. I encourage you and your partner(s) to be tested for all STDs before engaging in unprotected anal play. If you don't know your own status or that of your partner's, you should use safer sex barriers, like those discussed in chapter 6, to decrease the risk of infection transmission.

As women, we are the best source of information about our bodies, including our vaginas, clitorises, breasts, and butts. *You* know your body and its uniqueness better than anyone else. When you experience anything unusual—including bumps, rashes or sores, persistent itching, irritation, abdominal or pelvic pain, burning or pain during urination, any unusual discharge, irregular bleeding or cramping, or discomfort or pain during sex—you should see a gynecologist or other physician promptly. *For many women, STDs may occur without any symptoms at all*, so the only way they can be detected is through medical exams and laboratory tests. Therefore, all sexually active women should have checkups, pelvic exams, and pap smears on a yearly basis.

It is equally important to find a gynecologist or other physician you respect, trust, and feel comfortable talking to about your sexual health and practices. I've been to gynecologists who assume I'm heterosexual and ask me the requisite "What form of birth control do you use?" I've been to others who don't ask me anything about my sexual practices, partners, or concerns. Your gynecological visit is no time to play Don't Ask, Don't Tell. If they don't ask, it's your responsibility to tell. While a regular exam at the gynecologist can include a pelvic exam, pap smear, breast exam, and rectal exam, many doctors do not perform rectal exams unless patients specifically complain of symptoms related to their asses. If you regularly engage in anal sex of any kind, you should inform your doctor, be frank about your practices, and request a rectal exam, even if you feel fine. Sexually transmitted infections can be rectal as well as vaginal. If you are diagnosed with an STD in your pussy and have engaged in unprotected anal sex, make sure to get your ass tested as well. Because of the close proximity of our vaginas to our anuses, it is easy for women to spread infections from one orifice to the other. Most STDs can be treated and cured fairly easily with antibiotics or managed with other medications if they are caught in their early stages. Untreated STDs can lead to more serious complications, including sterility, cancer, and, in some cases, death. So please take care of yourself.

As in chapter 6, I will use the following terms and corresponding definitions, each of which assumes the unprotected form of sex (i.e., no safer sex barrier).

RUBBING: manual external stimulation with fingers, without penetration, without a glove.

FINGERING: anal penetration with a finger or fingers without a glove.

LICKING: analingus or rimming without a barrier.

ANAL INTERCOURSE: anal penetration with a penis, without a condom, with or without ejaculation.

SHARING SEX TOYS: transferring a sex toy from an infected person's orifice to another person's orifice without putting a condom on it or disinfecting it first.

Human Papillomavirus (HPV)

There are more than one hundred types of the human papillomavirus (HPV), and more than thirty different strains affect the genitals, including the ass. HPV is a virus most closely associated with genital or anal warts, although not all forms of HPV cause warts. Some of the strains are potentially cancerous including several that have been directly linked to cervical cancer. It is estimated that as many as one in ten people in the United States has HPV. You can spread HPV through anal intercourse, rubbing, fingering, licking, or sharing sex toys.

HPV often manifests itself as genital warts; however, in many cases, there are no external symptoms at all. Anal warts begin as small pink bumps that look like cauliflower florets around the anus and in the anal canal; they tend to spread rapidly, forming clumps of bumps that may be itchy. The bumps could be painful if they are irritated. Their incubation period is usually one to six months, but they can grow more rapidly if you are pregnant or have a compromised immune system.

HPV in the vagina can cause precancerous lesions on the cervix that can be detected through a pelvic exam and PAP test. If you have HPV in your ass, it's less common to have treatable precancerous lesions present since there is no cervix or cervix-like place for them to develop, though it's still possible to have pre-cancerous cells. If you have anal warts, a physician will be able to see them during a rectal exam with an anoscope. Anal warts are treated by removing them from the skin either through applying chemicals to them (usually acids), burning them with an electric needle (electrocautery), freezing them with liquid nitrogen (cryotherapy), or with laser treatment. Even after visible warts are removed, HPV remains in your body, and the anal warts can recur.

To test for the presence of HPV in the ass when there are no warts, a physician takes a swab of the rectum and sends it for laboratory analysis (similar to a vaginal PAP test). If you regularly engage in unprotected anal penetration and think you have been exposed to HPV, you can request a rectal exam and an anal papilloma screening (also known as an anal PAP test). The test can identify if there is HPV in and around the anus and anal canal; some people with HPV will never develop any symptoms, others may show precancerous cells which precede rectal cancer. You can spread HPV from your anus to your vagina and vice versa, so if it has been discovered in one place, it's advisable to get the other place checked. People diagnosed with HPV should have regular exams to monitor recurrences and prevent complications.

Genital Herpes

More than forty-five million people in the United States have been diagnosed with genital herpes. Most often genital herpes is caused by herpes simplex virus type 2 (HSV-2), as opposed to herpes simplex virus type 1 (HSV-1), the virus that causes oral herpes. Genital herpes is transmitted through sexual contact, including licking, anal intercourse, and, less commonly, rubbing or fingering with cuts in the skin and sharing sex toys.

Within a week of exposure, people with herpes usually first experience a tingly or burning sensation in the genital area; then they develop bumps,

Ask the Anal Advisor: *Genital Herpes*

Q: *My husband and I both already have genital herpes and were told not to bother with condoms now. He has recently become enamored with anal sex, but I want to know, can he spread the herpes virus there? Can you catch herpes when you already have it?*

A: Once you have the herpes virus, you have the antibodies in your system and cannot be reinfected. However, you didn't specify if you currently only have outbreaks in or around your vagina. You can spread genital herpes to other parts of the body. If your husband had an outbreak or was contagious but without symptoms and you had unprotected anal sex with him, he could pass the herpes virus to you rectally and cause you to have an outbreak in and around your ass. Then, you'd be prone to recurrent anal outbreaks. My guess is, if you've never had an outbreak anally, you don't want to start now, so a condom would be wise.

blisters, or open sores in the affected area, which can be itchy, sore, and/or painful. Women can also experience flu-like symptoms, swollen glands or lymph nodes, a vaginal discharge or yeast infection, and painful urination. Initial sores usually heal in one to three weeks without treatment.

There is no cure for herpes, and symptoms can recur during outbreaks. These outbreaks can be brought on by stress, a compromised immune system, or prolonged exposure to the sun; they can last for up to three weeks. Although a person is most contagious during an outbreak, transmission of the virus can happen during nonactive periods as well (especially the two weeks after an outbreak) and with or without visible blisters or other symptoms. Doctors prescribe medications like acyclovir, famiciclovir, or valacyclovir to both treat and prevent outbreaks, but there is no cure for genital herpes.[1]

Chlamydia

Chlamydia is a sexually transmitted bacterial infection and the most common STD in the United States. Seventy-five percent of women and fifty percent of men with chlamydia have no symptoms. It can be spread through anal intercourse, more rarely through sharing sex toys, rubbing or fingering if there are cuts in the skin, and very rarely (if ever) from licking. Common symptoms—if they do occur—can begin anywhere from five days to a few weeks after infection, and may include painful anal penetration, bowel movement discomfort, anal burning, soreness, and discharge; women may also experience swelling and soreness of the lymph nodes and rectal bleeding. Chlamydia is diagnosed through a rectal exam and treated with antibiotics like doxycycline and azithromycin.[2]

Gonorrhea

Rectal gonorrhea is a bacterial infection transmitted through different types of sexual contact including anal intercourse and licking, and less frequently, sharing sex toys, and rubbing or fingering if there are cuts in the skin. Symptoms appear within three to seven days of exposure and include soreness or burning during bowel movements and an anal discharge. Gonorrhea affects about 650,000 Americans every year. Up to 80 percent of women and about 10 percent of men who have gonorrhea have no symptoms; for women, this is even more true in cases of rectal gonorrhea than in those of vaginal gonorrhea. Rectal gonorrhea is treated with antibiotics, including penicillin, tetracycline, and ceftriaxone.

Syphilis

Much less common today than in the past—there are less than forty thousand reported cases in the United States—syphilis is a bacterial infection. Syphilis is transmitted by touching a sore on an infected person; sores can be on someone's mouth, penis, vagina, anus, or skin. You can spread it through anal intercourse, licking, rubbing or fingering (especially but not exclusively if there are cuts in the skin), and very rarely, sharing sex toys. Syphilis can have an incubation period of two to eight weeks. Ten to ninety days after exposure, people with syphilis experience the primary stage of the virus. A round ulcer (called a chancre) erupts in the affected area. The area in and around the chancre may ache or burn—or not. People may also have swollen lymph nodes. After the chancre hardens, heals, and disappears, the secondary stage begins. The secondary stage is marked by a general skin rash of sores the size of pennies that may be itchy and painful. You may also experience fever, swollen glands, aching joints, headaches, nausea, and/or constipation. This stage is when people are most contagious. The third and fourth stages, latent and tertiary, are very serious and can be deadly if untreated. Syphilis is treated with antibiotics, usually penicillin, doxycycline, or tetracycline.

Hepatitis A

Hepatitis A is an inflammation of the liver caused by the hepatitis A virus (HAV); the virus is transmitted when infected fecal matter gets into the mouth. A person who practices unprotected oral-anal sex *with an infected person and comes into contact with that person's fecal matter* is at risk. There are conflicting studies about how many cases of HAV are spread through sexual contact.

On average, the incubation period is thirty days, but can be anywhere from fourteen to sixty days. An individual is most infectious two weeks before and one week after he or she develops symptoms. Symptoms include fatigue, nausea, vomiting, abdominal pain, dark urine, light stools, fever, and jaundice (yellowing of the skin and eyes). You may become ill with several of these symptoms suddenly. Doctors can diagnose hepatitis A with a blood test. There is no treatment for hepatitis A, and it usually clears up on its own in weeks or months, depending on a person's immune system; the liver repairs itself and there is no permanent damage. Once you've had it, you develop antibodies for it and cannot have it again. In the United States, nearly one-hundred thousand new people contract HAV every year; there is a vaccine for the virus.[3]

Hepatitis B

The type of hepatitis most likely to be sexually transmitted is hepatitis B, an inflammatory liver disease caused by the hepatitis B virus (HBV). The virus is present in all bodily fluids of an infected person, including semen, saliva, vaginal secretions, blood, feces, menstrual blood, and sweat, although it can only be transmitted through blood, semen, and possibly saliva. It can be spread through anal intercourse and licking, and manual penetration if there is a cut on the skin and a tear in rectal tissue or rectal bleeding. *HBV is one hundred times easier to transmit sexually than HIV.* About eighty thousand Americans become infected with HBV each year. One out of twenty people in the United States will become infected with HBV sometime during their lives. Most of these infections occur among people who are twenty to forty-nine years old. There is an HBV vaccine to prevent hepatitis B that is given in multiple scheduled doses over four to six months.

About 50 percent of adults with HBV never have symptoms. When symptoms do occur, they appear between six weeks and six months after infection and may mimic flu symptoms: fatigue, nausea, vomiting, loss of appetite, headache, fever, tenderness and pain in the lower abdomen or joints, and possibly jaundice; more severe symptoms could be hives, severe abdominal pain, dark urine, and pale-colored bowel movements. Hepatitis B is diagnosed by a blood test.

About 95 percent of adults with hepatitis B develop antibodies to the virus and recover within two to six months without medication or treatment. While their blood will always test positive to the virus, they are immune and not infectious. The other 5 percent become chronically infected. They may or may not continue to show symptoms, but they will always be a carrier of the virus and can infect other people; they are at risk of developing cirrhosis, liver failure, and liver cancer. There are about 1.25 million HBV carriers in the United States. There is no treatment or cure for acute hepatitis B, but people with chronic hepatitis are prescribed different medications to eradicate or suppress the replication of the virus.[4]

Hepatitis C

Hepatitis C, also an inflammation of the liver, is caused by the hepatitis C virus (HCV). It is passed from person to person through direct contact with an infected person's blood. It is primarily spread through unsafe IV drug use, including sharing needles. Researchers disagree on the number of cases transmitted through sexual contact, and some studies "failed to detect the presence of HCV in either saliva, semen, or urine of HCV-infected people—except when those body fluids have been contaminated by the person's blood."[5] It may be spread through anal intercourse, but only when there are tears in the rectum or rectal bleeding and through fin-ger-fucking with rectal bleeding *and* cuts on the skin of the finger. HCV is more likely to be spread during sex if either of the sex partners also has HIV or another sexually transmitted disease.

Most infected people are asymptomatic or may have mild symptoms that resemble the flu: nausea, fatigue, loss of appetite, fever, headaches, and abdominal pain. Doctors do blood tests to determine if someone has HCV. Twenty to thirty percent of people can become disease-free with medication that contains the viral activity and reproduction and decreases inflammation in the liver. About 70–80 percent of people have chronic hepatitis C, and many of this group develop cirrhosis (scarring of the liver) or liver failure. There is no vaccine for HCV.[6]

HIV and AIDS

HIV, the virus that causes AIDS, is carried in and transmitted through bod-ily fluids and most concentrated in blood, semen, menstrual blood, breast milk, and vaginal secretions. HIV is transmitted in several ways: through unprotected sexual contact with the bodily fluids of an infected person, by sharing needles with an infected person (through intravenous drug use), by receiving infected blood (through a transfusion), or from mother to baby via amniotic fluid, during delivery or breast-feeding. It's easier for women to get AIDS from men through sexual intercourse than vice versa. The tis-sue of the vagina is more susceptible than the tissue of the penis to trauma, tears, and minute sores, which provide infected semen a direct route to the bloodstream. This is even more true of the tissue of the rectum, which is more delicate than that of the vagina. Plus, semen has a higher viral load than vaginal fluid, so infected semen is more infectious than infected vagi-nal secretions. Women and men can get the virus from anal intercourse, licking, and sharing toys, as well as from rubbing and fingering if there are cuts on the skin and in rectal tissue.

There is no cure for AIDS; however, there have been many advances in the treatment of the disease. With various combinations of prescription medications, people with HIV and AIDS are living longer, healthier lives now than in the past.

Anal Ailments

Many people assume that if you regularly engage in anal sex as the receptive partner, you are more likely to develop an anal ailment or disease. Myths abound about people having their rectums "stretched out" to the point of incontinence. As long as you practice safe, gradual anal penetration, you will not lose control of your bowels, no matter how often you do it. In fact, the opposite can be true: people who get buttfucked can have healthier asses than those who don't! It may sound surprising, but consider the facts: as you learn to relax and use your pelvic and sphincter muscles, you are exercising and toning them, just like any other muscle. Plus, the more awareness you have of those muscles and the more you practice relaxing them, the less likely you are to have recurring anal tension, difficult bowel movements, or problems like straining. During anal play, blood rushes to the area during arousal; this increases circulation, which is an important component for good anal health. The more you pay attention to your butt, the less alienated and anxious you will feel about it, so if something doesn't feel right, you'll be more likely to seek treatment sooner. With all that said, it is important to know about some of the common symptoms and ailments that involve your ass.

Constipation

After the food you eat passes through the digestive tract and your body has absorbed almost all the nutrients, what's left over enters the colon from the small intestine. The colon contracts to move the matter through as it absorbs nearly all the water from it; these contractions are controlled by nerves, hormones, and electrical activity in the colon muscle. After the water has been absorbed, what remains is the stool, which separates into segments, moves into the descending colon, then moves into the lower colon and rectum. The walls of the rectum expand, signaling to your brain that it's time to go to the bathroom. If you don't have a bowel movement right away or if the colon's contractions are slow, the colon continues to absorb more water from the stool. If it absorbs too much water, the stool becomes hard and compact and splits into smaller pieces. This causes constipation: difficult or painful bowel movements that may be accompanied by bloating and discomfort. The most common causes of constipation are not enough fiber in your diet, dehydration, lack of exercise, and stress; it can also be caused by pregnancy, certain medications, and old age. Mild constipation usually rectifies itself or can be alleviated by the use of natural remedies or over-the-counter laxatives. Chronic constipation may be a sign of a more serious problem.

If you are constipated, chances are you don't feel like having something in your ass, but know that anal penetration does not cause, nor should it exacerbate, constipation. In fact, some medical professionals admit that anal play may in fact help to "move things along." Remember that the contractions of the pelvic muscles experienced during anal sex are similar to the contractions during a bowel movement (that's why sometimes when you're penetrated you feel like you have to go). Anal stimulation may help the rectum relax, and repeated anal sessions may improve circulation and decrease tension in the entire area.

Diarrhea

As waste moves through the colon, if the colon does not absorb the majority of the water, you have the opposite of constipation, which is diarrhea: loose or runny stools. They may be accompanied by cramping, bloating, nausea, fatigue, and fever. Acute diarrhea (diarrhea that lasts for a short time) is most often caused by a bacteria, virus, or parasite getting into your digestive tract and inhibiting the colon's ability to absorb water. Most people come into contact with it from uncooked, undercooked, or spoiled food. You can be exposed to it through food that has been contaminated with fecal matter by food handlers who didn't properly wash their hands after going to the bathroom. You can also come into contact with a bacteria, virus, or parasite in someone's fecal matter through anal contact, specifically rimming or ass-to-mouth play: transferring a cock that's been in someone's ass directly to his or her mouth. Intestinal disease or conditions like Irritable Bowel Syndrome can also cause chronic diarrhea, which is not related to an infection and therefore cannot be passed person to person. If you have diarrhea, it's important to drink plenty of fluids to keep your body hydrated. Diarrhea should go away on its own without special treatment, although you can use over the counter products to treat symptoms. If it lasts for more than three days and is accompanied by a high fever or bloody stools, you should see a doctor.

While anal penetration doesn't cause diarrhea, it can sometimes make your body more susceptible to loose or runny bowel movements. After a vigorous round of anal penetration complete with plenty of lube, some of the lube will be absorbed by the body, but the rest of it will come out in the toilet. Rarely, but for some people, anal penetration can stimulate an early bowel movement; by early, I don't mean right there in the middle of things. But soon after sex, you'll feel the need to expel. Since the bowel movement is premature, the colon has not had a chance to absorb all the water before the stool moves into the rectum, and this will cause diarrhea. In both cases, you should be back to normal within twenty-four hours.

Hemorrhoids

Hemorrhoids are the most common of all anal ailments, and it is estimated that nearly half of all adults have them by the age of fifty. Hemorrhoids occur when blood vessels in the anal canal or around the anus fill with blood and form tiny sacs that become swollen and inflamed. This engorgement is caused by pressure on the vessels, which can happen as a result of constipation, straining, or diarrhea. Hemorrhoids can also be caused by pregnancy, sitting or standing for long periods of time, and even heavy lifting. Hemorrhoids can be internal or external, and may cause itching, swelling, discomfort, bleeding, and pain. External hemorrhoids are those found just inside the anal opening; as the blood vessels swell, they can actually protrude during bowel movements or become so large that they protrude all the time. If a blood clot forms, a hard bump can be created and be very painful. The most common symptom of an internal hemorrhoid is bleeding: bright red blood in your stool or on the toilet paper when you wipe.

The treatment for hemorrhoids depends on their severity. In mild cases, the body heals itself, symptoms go away in a few days, and the hemorrhoid shrinks. If the hemorrhoid is a result of the diet, adding more fiber helps regulate bowel movements. Most people use over-the-counter creams and ointments and take warm baths to relieve symptoms. There are also many herbal and homeopathic remedies, including aloe vera and slippery elm (taken orally or used topically). If you have chronic or painful hemorrhoids, you should see a doctor. There are several kinds of treatments to shrink or remove more serious hemorrhoids. In rubber band ligation, a band is placed around the base of the hemorrhoid, it is deprived of blood, and it dies and falls off. Chemical injections and laser treatments are used to shrink hemorrhoids. Hemorrhoids may also be surgically removed, but that is only recommended in very severe cases.

Anal penetration does not cause hemorrhoids; however, it may irritate them, especially if you don't use enough lube or you rupture a blood-filled vessel. The general rule is to listen to your body—if you are having a flare-up and experience itching or discomfort, you may want to take a break from anal play until symptoms subside. Going in is often fine, but coming out can be much more irritating, especially to external hemorrhoids. If that's the case, you may want to opt for a butt plug or more gentle motion rather than lots of in-and-out action. I'd also recommend using smooth toys versus those with balls, ridges, bumps, and other stimulating textures.

Anal Fissures

An anal fissure is a cut in the tissue of the anus, anal canal, or rectum. Fissures are usually the result of some kind of trauma to the ass—like penetration without lubrication or proper warm-up. Penetration with a sex toy with rough edges or seams (common in cheaply made toys), digital penetration with a jagged fingernail, or severe constipation can also cause a fissure. The lining of the anal canal and rectum is delicate and even with the most gentle touch, sometimes we can tear the tissue slightly and not even know it or feel any pain. Most fissures are internal and therefore not visible; the symptoms are pain and minor bleeding. If you suspect you have a fissure, you should give your ass a vacation from penetration and other play until your symptoms subside, both to help it heal and because lube will likely irritate it. Your body should heal itself without treatment, although you may want to take warm baths or use witch hazel wipes if the cut is external. If your symptoms last for more than a few days, you should see a physician.

At the first sight of blood coming from their asses, most people become alarmed. It's only natural. If you see a small amount of bright red blood in the toilet after a postsex bowel movement or on the tissue when you wipe yourself, chances are there is no real cause for panic. If, however, there is more than just a little blood, the blood is dark red or brown, the bleeding persists for more than a few days, or you have other symptoms with the bleeding, then you should see a doctor. Bleeding and blood in the stool can be a symptom of more serious diseases, including ulcers, gastritis, ulcerative colitis, Crohn's disease, polyps, diverticulitis, anal fistula, an abscess, or a sexually transmitted infection.

Irritable Bowel Syndrome (IBS)

Irritable Bowel Syndrome (IBS) is a disorder that affects how the colon works. As discussed previously in this chapter, in a healthy person, food is digested and nutrients are absorbed by the body, then the remaining matter enters the colon where most of the water is absorbed. For people with IBS, the colon seems to be more sensitive to food, stress, and other elements. As a result, it may contract (and move matter through it) too fast or too slow and thus absorb too much or too little water. People with IBS experience chronic bouts of constipation or diarrhea or both and have a range of symptoms associated with those conditions, including cramps, bloating, abdominal discomfort, nausea, and fatigue.

According to the National Institutes of Health, one in five Americans has IBS, and it affects women much more than men. IBS can be treated in several ways: with changes in diet, exercise, and stress reduction; with over-the-counter or prescription medications that treat constipation and diarrhea; or with a combination of these. There is no cure, nor one kind of treatment.

If you have IBS, chances are you're pretty in touch with the nuances of your bowel movements. When symptoms are at their worst, anal sex is probably the last thing on your mind. IBS does not prevent you from having a fulfilling anal sex life, it may just cause it to be a less frequent one. The guidelines for constipation and diarrhea apply to those with IBS as well. Listen to your body: if it feels okay, then you're not doing any harm. Also talk to your doctor about his or her recommendations.[7]

Anal Wellness

The better your ass feels, the more likely you'll want to engage in anal play; that's a no-brainer, right? Well, our asses can say a lot about our overall health, too. If we are overworked, tense, exhausted, nervous, tired, depressed, or sick, our butts will often manifest these states by being out of whack. Symptoms may disappear as we exercise, eat well, decrease stress, and achieve better balance in our lives. Or they may not go away on their own and be the sign of something serious. Listen to your body, use common sense, and see your doctor if you are concerned.

Ask the Anal Advisor: *Urinary Tract Infections*

Q: *I develop a urinary tract infection almost every time I have anal sex, and it is really frustrating. I thought I was doing everything right. I have an enema beforehand. I make sure there is not too much fondling of my vagina during anal sex (although I hate that, as I always enjoy his fingers or a toy inside me during anal). We do not switch from tushy to pussy, and my ass is almost always very clean, although I realize that we can only be so clean, as there is microscopic bacteria in the rectum. I would appreciate any recommendations you have, so I can stop having urinary tract infections and keep having more anal sex.*

A: Many women get urinary tract infections (UTIs) after sex because bacteria from your partner's cock or your ass gets into the urethra, where it causes an infection. It sounds to me like you may be especially prone to UTIs if you are getting them so frequently. You have been doing all the right things (enema, no ass to pussy, no vaginal play during anal) to prevent a possible infection, but I do have some additional advice. First and foremost, make sure that lube from your ass isn't "migrating" to your pussy. This is a common problem, especially if you are doing it doggie-style. One way to prevent what I call "the drip down effect" is to switch to a different position, like missionary, where gravity is working in your favor. You should also try to keep some unscented baby wipes on hand to wipe excess lube away from your butt before it makes its way to your pussy. After sex, the first thing you should do is pee, even if you feel like you don't have to. The simple act of urinating can flush out any bacteria that may have gotten into your urethra. Then, shower to wash away lube, semen, and any other body fluids you've got in or on you. Use castile soap, which is gentler on the genitals than traditional bar soap or body wash. Make sure you drink plenty of water after anal sex, to help flush bacteria and other toxins from the body and clear out the urethra.

NOTES

1. "Genital Herpes," by Jon Knowles (1989), updated by Jennifer Johnsen and Jessica Davis (December 2004), www.plannedparenthood.org.

2. "Chlamydia," by Jon Knowles, revised by Jennifer Johnsen (March 2004), www.planned-parenthood.org.

3. *Dr. Palmer's Guide to Hepatitis and Liver Disease,* by Melissa Palmer, M.D. (Avery, 2004) 82; Hepatitis Foundation International, www.hepfi.org.

4. Palmer, 92, 93; "Hepatitis B," by Danielle Dimitrov (February 2004), www.plannedpar-enthood.org; Hepatitis Foundation International, www.hepfi.org.

5. Palmer, 114.

6. Palmer, 114; Hepatitis Foundation International, www.hepfi.org

7. "Irritable Bowel Syndrome," (April 2003), National Digestive Disease Information Clearinghouse (NDDIC), a service of the National Institute of Diabetes and Digestive and Kidney Diseases (NIDDK), National Institutes of Health, www.digestive.niddk.nih.gov.

CHAPTER 18

The Ultimate Frontier

My goal for this book is to give people, especially women, knowledge about their bodies, so we may all have safe, pleasurable anal erotic experiences. Before I wrote the first edition, I came across plenty of women who really enjoy anal sex—the unique physical sensations, the emotional intensity, the complex psychological dynamics. These same women took a major step in breaking their silence to tell me that they love anal sex. Then they told me why they love to do it, how they love to do it, when they love do it, and with whom (or what) they love to do it. It felt great to finally hear other women's stories and not feel so alone with my own desires, fantasies, and experiences of anal sex. I hoped *The Ultimate Guide to Anal Sex for Women* would incite this kind of communication among its readers and the dialogue would continue. Boy did it ever.

I'm thrilled by the response to the book, and I'm excited that I had so much more to say the second time around. And I hope there's more to come—more scientific, medical, and anecdotal research; more surveys; more books. Just think: the more information we have, the more anal sex we can have!

If you picked up this book, you have some desire and curiosity to learn more about anal sexuality. If you've gotten this far, my desire is that you will now be armed with information, resources, ideas, and some answers to your questions. Use this book with love, understanding, desire, and trust; ideally, it will reward you with some hot, sexy anal play. Remember that patience and practice make perfect. In my anal erotic experiences, I've felt sheer bliss, absolute surrender, indescribable rapture, and overwhelming pleasure—and I haven't gotten anywhere near perfect yet. In fact, I don't really want to. For me, the ultimate thrill is in the voyage.

CHAPTER 19

Resource Guide

Books

Anal Pleasure and Health by Jack Morin, Ph.D. (San Francisco: Down There Press, 1998).

Basic In-Home Colon Cleansing: An Illustrated Guide (CD-ROM) by Edith Webber (Health Management Research Institute, 2003).

The Clitoral Truth by Rebecca Chalker (New York: Seven Stories Press, 2000).

Dr. Jensen's Guide to Better Bowel Care by Bernard Jensen (New York: Avery Publishing Group, 1998).

The Enema as an Erotic Art and Its History by David Barton-Jay (David Barton-Jay Projects, 1984).

The Erotic Mind: Unlocking the Inner Sources of Sexual Passion and Fulfillment by Jack Morin (New York: HarperCollins, 1995).

Female Ejaculation and the G-Spot by Deborah Sundahl (Alameda, CA: Hunter House, 2003).

The First Year: Hepatitis B—An Essential Guide for the Newly Diagnosed by William Finley Green (New York: Marlowe & Company, 2002).

The First Year: Hepatitis C—An Essential Guide for the Newly Diagnosed by Cara Bruce and Lisa Montanarelli (New York: Marlowe & Company, 2002).

The Good Vibrations Guide to Sex by Cathy Winks and Anne Semans (San Francisco: Cleis Press, 2002).

Guide to Getting It On by Paul Joannides (Chicago: Goofy Foot Press, 2004).

Intimate Invasions: The Erotic Ins and Outs of Enema Play by M. R. Strict (Oakland, CA: Greenery Press, 2004).

Love Thine Enemas & Heal Thyself by Dr. Jerry Glenn Knox (Vancouver, WA: Lifeknox Publishing, 2002).

The Many Joys of Sex Toys by Anne Semans (New York: Broadway Books, 2004).

Orgasms for Two: The Joy of Partnersex by Betty Dodson, Ph.D. (New York: Harmony Books, 2002).

Screw the Roses, Send Me the Thorns: The Romance and Sexual Sorcery of Sadomasochism by Phillip Miller and Molly Devon (Fairfield, CT: Mystic Rose Books, 1995).

Sex for One: The Joy of Selfloving by Betty Dodson (New York: Three Rivers Press, 1996).

Sex Toys 101: A Playfully Uninhibited Guide by Rachel Venning and Claire Cavanah (New York: Fireside Books, 2003).

SM 101: A Realistic Introduction by Jay Wiseman (Oakland, CA: Greenery Press, 1998).

The Surrender: An Erotic Memoir by Toni Bentley (New York: ReganBooks, 2004).

Trust: The Hand Book—A Guide to the Sensual and Spiritual Art of Hand-balling by Bert Herrman (San Francisco: Alamo Square Press, 1991).

The Ultimate Guide to Anal Sex for Men by Bill Brent (San Francisco: Cleis Press, 2002).

The Ultimate Guide to Strap-on Sex by Karlyn Lotney (San Francisco: Cleis Press, 2000).

Enema Equipment and Information

Arthur Hamilton Inc., www.arthurhamilton.com, 888-783-6937
In business since 1972 when he did mail-order catalogs, Arthur Hamilton is finally on the Web with a great selection of enema equipment, including double inflatable nozzles, the hard-to-find pumpkin bag, larger bags, the sit-on bag, and stands.

Beth Tyler Labs, www.bethtyler.com, 972-772-9393
The best online selection of all things enema at reasonable prices, including double inflatable nozzles, silicone bags and tubing, and hard-to-find exclusive designs, plus there is a membership component to this site with message boards, stories, photos, and videos.

Enema Bag, www.enemabag.com
Large selection of enema supplies plus good enema education and health information.

Enema Lovers Guide, www.enemaloversguide.com
Great resource with lots of links to other enema websites.

Klystra, www.klystra.com
Manufacturer and retailer of enema supplies including rectal dilators.

Shopping Guide

665 Leather and Fetish Company, www.665leather.com, 310-854-7276
    722 Santa Monica Blvd., West Hollywood, CA 90069
    Retail and online store specializing in leather that carries anal toys,
    butt plug harnesses, enema equipment, inflatable toys, J-Lube, shower
    attachment equipment, and slings.

Adam and Eve, www.adameve.com, 800-274-0333
    Mail-order and online store with toys, videos, and lingerie.

Aneros, www.aneros.com
    Makers of the unique prostate massage toy.

Astroglide/Paradise Marketing, www.paradisemarketing.com
    Makers of Astroglide Gel and Astroglide Gel Shooters.

A Woman's Touch, www.a-womans-touch.com, 888-621-8880
    600 Williamson St., Madison, WI 53703
    Women-owned and -run retail and online store with toys, books,
    videos, and safer sex supplies.

Babeland, www.babeland.com, 800-658-9119
    707 E. Pike St., Seattle, WA 98122
    94 Rivington St., New York, NY 10002
    43 Mercer St., New York, NY 10013
    7007 Melrose Ave., Los Angeles, CA 90038
    Sex-positive, women-owned retail and online store with toys, books,
    videos, and safer sex supplies.

Blowfish, www.blowfish.com, 800-325-2569
    Sex-positive mail-order and online store with toys, books, videos, and
    a small selection of enema equipment, including anodized aluminum
    butt plug nozzles and shower shot kit.

Bungee Sexperience, www.bungeesex.com, 702-260-7475
Makers of the Bungee Sexperience sex swing.

Come As You Are, www.comeasyouare.com, 877-858-3160
701 Queen St. W, Toronto, Ontario, Canada M6J 1E6
Sex-positive retail and online store with toys, books, videos, and safer sex supplies.

Cottonballs.com
Online drugstore that carries lube, Fleet enemas, as well as latex, vinyl, nitrile, and neoprene/chloroprene gloves.

Early 2 Bed, www.early2bed.com, 773-271-1219
5232 N. Sheridan, Chicago, IL 60640
Sex-positive retail and online store with toys, books, videos, and safer sex supplies.

Eros Boutique, www.erosboutique.com, 866-425-0345
581A Tremont St., Boston, MA 02118
Retail and online store; carries anal toys, butt plug harnesses, chrome syringes, enema equipment, inflatable enema nozzles, Liberator Shapes, unique anal toys, and swings.

Eve's Garden, www.evesgarden.com, 800-848-3837
119 W. 57th St., 12th Floor, New York, NY 10019
Established in 1972, a sex-positive retail and online store that caters to women and carries toys, books, videos, and safer sex supplies.

EQ+, www.eqplus.com, 800-771-1218
Medical supply website that carries latex, nitrile, and vinyl gloves.

Extreme Restraints, www.extremerestraints.com, 866-4MY-BDSM
Online store specializing in BDSM toys that carries enema equipment, inflatable toys, J-Lube, slings, swings, and unique anal toys.

Fisher Scientific, www.fishersci.com, 800-766-7000
    Medical supply website that carries latex (regular and extra long), nitrile (regular and extra long), vinyl, neoprene/chloroprene (regular and extra long), polyethylene (regular and extra long) and other nonlatex gloves; U.S. orders only.

Forbidden Fruit, www.forbiddenfruit.com, 800-315-2029
    512 Neches, Austin, TX 78701
    Sex-positive retail and online store with toys, books, videos, and safer sex supplies.

Good for Her, www.goodforher.com, 416-588-0900
    175 Harbord St., Toronto, Ontario, Canada M5S 1H3
    Sex-positive, women-owned and -run retail and online store that carries toys, books, videos, and safer sex supplies.

Good Vibrations, www.goodvibes.com, 800-289-8423
    603 Valencia St., San Francisco, CA 94110
    1620 Polk St., San Francisco, CA 94109
    2504 San Pablo Ave., Berkeley, CA 94702
    Sex-positive, worker-owned retail and online stores with toys, books, videos, and safer sex supplies.

Grand Opening! Sexuality Boutique, www.grandopening.com, 877-731-262
    308A Harvard St., Brookline, MA 02446
    Sex-positive, women-owned retail and online store with toys, books, videos, and safer sex supplies.

Grogans, www.grogans.com, 800-365-1020
    Medical supply website that carries latex (regular and extra long), nitrile, and neoprene/chloroprene gloves (regular and extra long).

Innerspace, www.innerspace1.com
    Online home of Ray Cirino, designer and manufacturer of unique acrylic and metal toys, including clear acrylic butt plugs.

It's My Pleasure, 503-236-0505
4258 SE Hawthorne Blvd., Portland, OR 97215
Sex-positive, women-owned retail store with toys, books, videos, and safer sex supplies.

J-Lube, www.jlube.net
Comprehensive information about J-Lube.

JT's Stockroom, www.stockroom.com, 800-755-TOYS
Sex-positive mail-order and online store with toys, books, videos, safer sex supplies, slings, swings, BDSM gear, enema supplies, anal speculums, and butt plug harnesses.

Kinky Medical, www.kinkymedical.net
Online store that carries latex and nitrile gloves, extra-long latex gloves, J-Lube and J-Jelly, stainless steel syringes, enema supplies, and other medical equipment.

Liberator Shapes, www.liberatorshapes.com
Makers of a unique brand of firm, supportive shapes that help to angle the body better for sex.

Libida, www.libida.com
Sex-positive online store that caters to women and carries toys, books, videos, and safer sex supplies.

Love Swing, www.loveswing.com, 541-261-6656
Makers of the Love Swing.

Lube Shooter, www.lubeshooter.com
Makers of plastic disposable lube shooters.

Medical Toys, www.medicaltoys.com, 800-791-3931
Online store that carries anal toys, stainless steel enema/lube syringes, enema equipment, and anal speculums.

MFASCO Health & Safety, www.mfasco.com, 800-221-9222
Medical supply website that carries latex (regular and extra long), nitrile, and vinyl gloves.

Midnight Blue's, www.midnight-blues.net
Online store specializing in BDSM toys that carries a good selection of unique inflatable rubber toys.

Miko Exoticwear, www.mikoexoticwear.com, 800-421-6646
653 N. Main St., Providence, RI 02904
Retail and online store with toys, books, videos, and safer sex supplies, including good selection of anal toys and the chrome syringe.

Mr. S Leather, www.mr-s-leather.com, 800-SHOP-MRS
310 Seventh St., San Francisco, CA 94103
Retail and online store specializing in BDSM toys that carries butt plug harnesses, enema equipment, inflatable toys, unique anal toys, and slings.

Purple Passion, www.purplepassion.com, 212-807-0486
211 W. 20th St., New York, NY 10011
Retail and online store specializing in BDSM toys and clothing that carries anal toys, butt plug harnesses, and inflatable toys.

Rainbow Rope, www.rainbowrope.com
Online store specializing in BDSM toys that carries latex and nitrile gloves, stainless steel syringes, enema equipment, rubber and silicone double balloon nozzles, latex tubing in a rainbow of colors, plastic irrigation syringes, anal scopes and speculums.

Shop in Private, www.shopinprivate.com
Online store that carries enemas, some enema equipment, condoms, lube, and anal bleaching cream.

The Smitten Kitten, www.smittenkittenonline.com, 888-751-0523
3010 Lyndale Ave. S, Minneapolis, MN 55408
Sex-positive, women-owned retail and online store with toys, books, videos, and safer sex supplies.

Stormy Leather, www.stormyleather.com, 800-486-9650
1158 Howard St., San Francisco, CA 94103
Sex-positive retail and online store that specializes in leather and latex fetishwear, manufactures some of the best dildo harnesses, and also carries some toys, books, videos, and safer sex supplies.

The Toy Bag, www.toybag.com
Online store specializing in BDSM toys that carries hand-tooled hardwood dildos and bead toys.

Venus Envy, www.venusenvy.ca, 877-370-9288
1598 Barrington St., Halifax, Nova Scotia, Canada B3J 1Z6
110 Parent Ave., Ottawa, Ontario, Canada K1N 7B4
Sex-positive retail and online store with toys, books, videos, and safer sex supplies.

Vixen Creations, www.vixencreations.com
Women-owned and run sex toy manufacturer and retailer.

Whirlwind, www.brownbottle.com, 866-744-8697
Online store that carries anal toys, lube, stainless steel enema/lube syringes, enema equipment, anal spreaders, anal scopes, slings, other BDSM products.

Womyns' Ware, www.womynsware.com, 888-WYM-WARE
896 Commercial Dr., Vancouver, BC Canada V5L 3Y5
Sex-positive retail and online store that caters to women and carries toys, books, videos, and safer sex supplies.

Videos

Anal Massage for Lovers directed and produced by Joseph Kramer and EROSpirit Institute, 2005, 130 minutes. Available at www.eroticmassage.com and sex-positive stores.

Anal Massage for Relaxation and Pleasure directed and produced by Joseph Kramer and EROSpirit Institute, 2004, 160 minutes. Available at www.eroticmassage.com and sex-positive stores.

Bend Over Boyfriend directed by Shar Rednour, produced by Fatale Video, 1998, 60 minutes. Available at www.fatalemedia.com, 888-5-FATALE, and most sex-positive stores.

Bend Over Boyfriend 2: More Rockin', Less Talkin' directed by Shar Rednour and Jackie Strano, produced by S.I.R. Video, 1999, 70 minutes. Available at sirvideo.com and most sex-positive stores.

College Guide to Anal Sex, produced by Shane's World Productions, 2004. Available at videos stores.

Handball Loving directed by Gene Hubris, produced by Bert Herrman's Alamo Square, 35 minutes. Available at www.bijouworld.com and other websites (hard to find).

Nina Hartley's Guide to Anal Sex directed by Nina Hartley, produced by Adam & Eve, 1996, 70 minutes. Available at www.adameve.com and most sex-positive stores.

Tristan Taormino's House of Ass directed by Tristan Taormino, produced by Adam & Eve, 2006, 140 minutes. Available at www.puckerup.com and most sex-positive stores.

Tristan Taormino's Ultimate Guide to Anal Sex for Women directed and produced by Tristan Taormino, Ernest Greene, and John Stagliano, 1999, 238 minutes. Available at www.puckerup.com and most sex-positive stores.

Tristan Taormino's Ultimate Guide to Anal Sex for Women 2 directed and produced by Tristan Taormino and Ernest Greene, 2001, 135 minutes. Available at www.puckerup.com and most sex-positive stores.

Websites

Betty Dodson, www.bettydodson.com
　　Author, masturbation guru, sex educator, producer of self-loving videos.

Planned Parenthood, www.ppfa.org
　　STD and safer sex information.

Red Right, www.winternet.com/%7Eredright/redright.html
　　Anal fisting information and resources.

San Francisco Sex Information, www.sfsi.org, 415-989-SFSI
　　Free information and referral switchboard providing anonymous, accurate, nonjudgmental information about sex.

Susie Bright, www.susiebright.com
　　Author, sexpert.

Violet Blue, www.tinynibbles.com
　　Author, oral sex expert, sex educator.

Index

About the Author

TRISTAN TAORMINO is the author of *True Lust: Adventures in Sex, Porn and Perversion* and *Down and Dirty Sex Secrets*. She is series editor of all thirteen volumes of *Best Lesbian Erotica,* two of which have won Lambda Literary Awards. She is director, producer, and star of two videos based on her book, *Tristan Taormino's Ultimate Guide to Anal Sex for Women 1* and *2,* the first of which won two Adult Video News Awards in 2000. She returns to the world of adult video in 2006 as director and producer of *Tristan Taormino's House of Ass,* which will be released by Adam & Eve Pictures. She is the sex columnist for the *Village Voice,* a columnist for *Taboo* and *Velvetpark,* and the former editor of *On Our Backs.* Tristan has been featured in over two hundred publications including the *New York Times, Redbook, Cosmopolitan, Glamour, New York Magazine, Men's Health,* and *Playboy.* She has been named to several media lists, including *Out Magazine's* "100 Gay Success Stories of the Year" and *The Advocate's* "Best and Brightest Gay & Lesbian People Under 30." She has appeared on CNN, MSNBC, HBO's *Real Sex,* NBC's *The Other Half, The Howard Stern Show, Loveline, Ricki Lake,* MTV, Oxygen, Fox News, The Discovery Channel, and on dozens of radio shows. She lectures at top colleges and universities including Yale, Brown, Columbia, Smith, Vassar, and NYU, where she speaks on gay and lesbian issues, sexuality and gender, and feminism. She teaches sex and relationship workshops around the world and does private coaching sessions for individuals and couples. She lives with her partner and their three dogs in New York City. Her official website is www.puckerup.com.

About the Illustrator

FISH likes drawing, bicycling, tattooing, fucking, crafting, and queering up the world. Right now she's in the sculpture program at the California College of the Arts, finally finishing an undergrad degree after twenty years of the above. Her tattoo portfolio and art projects are online at www.devilfish.com.